Contents

Art school confidential — iv

Contributors and consultants — vi

1 The human body — 1

2 Genetics — 19

3 Chemical organization — 25

4 Integumentary system — 35

5 Musculoskeletal system — 43

6 Nervous system — 57

7 Sensory system — 71

8 Endocrine system — 81

9 Cardiovascular system — 93

10 Hematologic system — 107

11 Immune system — 117

12 Respiratory system — 133

13 Gastrointestinal system — 151

14 Nutrition and metabolism — 171

15 Urinary system — 191

16 Fluids, electrolytes, acids, and bases — 201

17 Reproductive system — 213

18 Reproduction and lactation — 225

Selected references — 243

Credits — 244

Index — 245

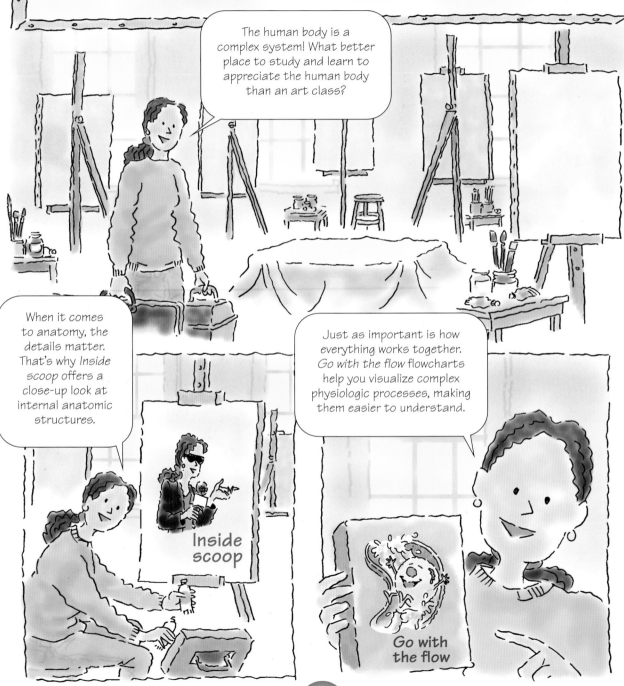

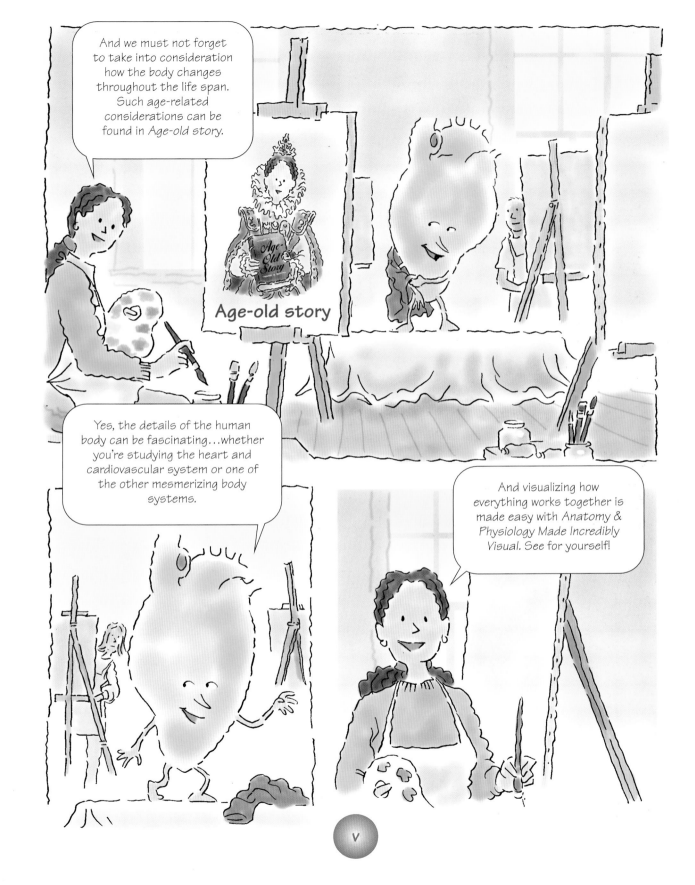

Contributors and consultants

Helen C. Ballestas, RN, MS, CRRN
Nursing Faculty
New York Institute of Technology
Old Westbury

James S. Davis IV, RN, BSN, CCRN
Infection Control Practitioner
Abington (Pa.) Memorial Hospital

Collette Bishop Hendler, RN, MS, CCRN
Infection Control Nurse
Abington (Pa.) Memorial Hospital

Fiona Johnson, RN, BS, MSN, CCRN
Clinical Education Specialist
Memorial Health University Medical
  Center
Savannah, Ga.

Jennifer M. Lee, FNP-C, MSN, CCRN
Nurse Practitioner
Greenville (S.C.) Hospital System –
  Pulmonary Disease Associates

Marilyn D. Sellers, APRN,BC, MS, FNP
Family Nurse Practitioner –
  Environmental/Compensation &
  Pension Clinician
Veterans Administration Medical Center
Hampton, Va.

Allison J. Terry, RN, MSN, PhD
Director, Center for Nursing
Alabama Board of Nursing
Montgomery

Leigh Ann Trujillo, RN, BSN
Nurse Educator
St. James Hospital & Health Centers
Olympia Fields, Ill.

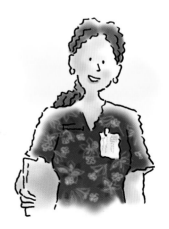

1
The human body

Anatomic terms 2
Cells 6
Tissue 14
Vision quest 18

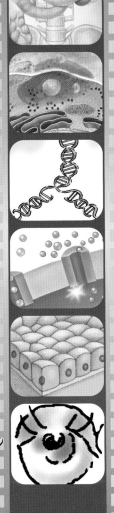

Let's get this show started. Seeing the big picture is the first step toward understanding anatomy and physiology.

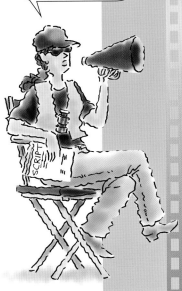

Anatomic terms

Knowing the anatomic terms for direction, reference planes, body cavities, and body regions will help you navigate the body's various structures.

Directional terms

Generally, directional terms can be grouped into pairs of opposites.

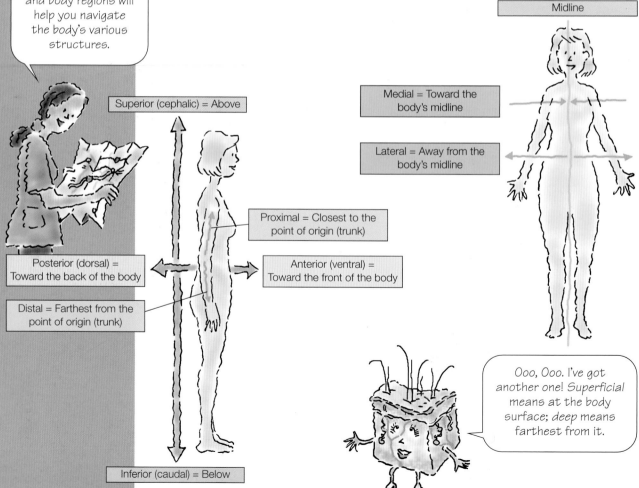

Midline

Medial = Toward the body's midline

Lateral = Away from the body's midline

Superior (cephalic) = Above

Proximal = Closest to the point of origin (trunk)

Posterior (dorsal) = Toward the back of the body

Anterior (ventral) = Toward the front of the body

Distal = Farthest from the point of origin (trunk)

Inferior (caudal) = Below

Ooo, Ooo. I've got another one! *Superficial* means at the body surface; *deep* means farthest from it.

Reference planes

Reference planes are imaginary lines used to section the body and its organs. These lines run longitudinally, horizontally, and on an angle.

Oh boy! Anatomical planes that aren't parallel to sagittal, frontal, or transverse planes are termed *oblique planes*.

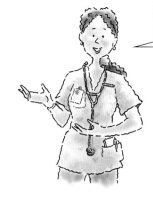

Median sagittal

The median sagittal plane passes through the center of the body, dividing it into two equal right and left halves.

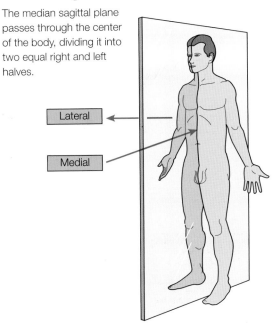

Lateral

Medial

Frontal

The frontal plane, also called the *coronal plane,* passes at a right angle to the medial plane, dividing the body into front and back portions.

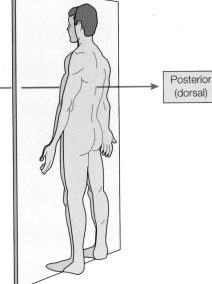

Anterior (ventral)

Posterior (dorsal)

Transverse

The transverse, or horizontal, plane is at a right angle to both the median and frontal planes; it divides the body into upper and lower sections.

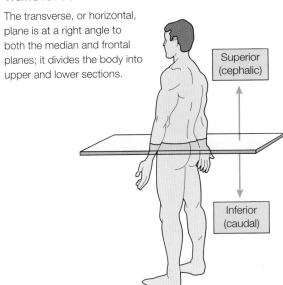

Superior (cephalic)

Inferior (caudal)

Body cavities

Body cavities are spaces within the body that contain internal organs. The dorsal and ventral cavities are the two major closed cavities—cavities without direct openings to the outside of the body.

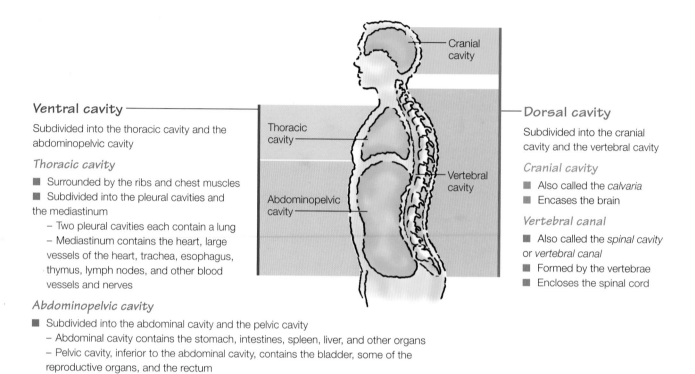

Ventral cavity

Subdivided into the thoracic cavity and the abdominopelvic cavity

Thoracic cavity

■ Surrounded by the ribs and chest muscles
■ Subdivided into the pleural cavities and the mediastinum
  – Two pleural cavities each contain a lung
  – Mediastinum contains the heart, large vessels of the heart, trachea, esophagus, thymus, lymph nodes, and other blood vessels and nerves

Abdominopelvic cavity

■ Subdivided into the abdominal cavity and the pelvic cavity
  – Abdominal cavity contains the stomach, intestines, spleen, liver, and other organs
  – Pelvic cavity, inferior to the abdominal cavity, contains the bladder, some of the reproductive organs, and the rectum

Dorsal cavity

Subdivided into the cranial cavity and the vertebral cavity

Cranial cavity

■ Also called the *calvaria*
■ Encases the brain

Vertebral canal

■ Also called the *spinal cavity* or *vertebral canal*
■ Formed by the vertebrae
■ Encloses the spinal cord

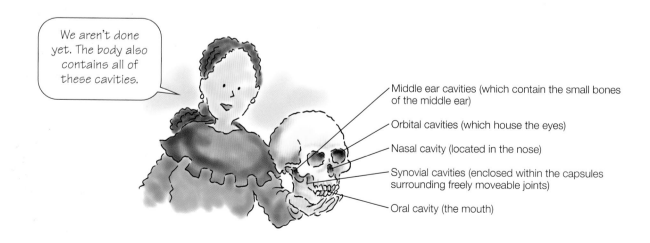

We aren't done yet. The body also contains all of these cavities.

Middle ear cavities (which contain the small bones of the middle ear)

Orbital cavities (which house the eyes)

Nasal cavity (located in the nose)

Synovial cavities (enclosed within the capsules surrounding freely moveable joints)

Oral cavity (the mouth)

Body regions

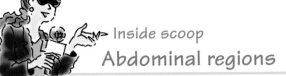

Inside scoop

Abdominal regions

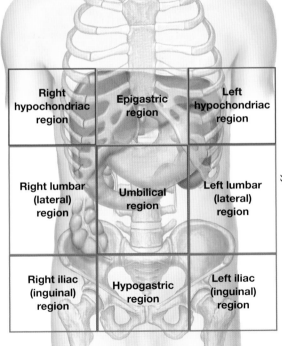

Right hypochondriac region	Epigastric region	Left hypochondriac region
Right lumbar (lateral) region	Umbilical region	Left lumbar (lateral) region
Right iliac (inguinal) region	Hypogastric region	Left iliac (inguinal) region

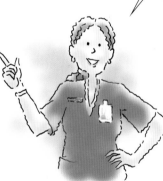

Body regions identify areas that have a special nerve or vascular supply or those that perform a special function. The most widely used terms designate regions in the abdomen.

Right and left hypochondriac
■ Contain the diaphragm, portions of the kidneys, the right side of the liver, the spleen, and part of the pancreas

Epigastric
■ Contains most of the pancreas and portions of the stomach, liver, inferior vena cava, abdominal aorta, and duodenum

Right and left lumbar (lateral)
■ Include portions of the small and large intestines and portions of the kidneys

Umbilical
■ Includes sections of the small and large intestines, inferior vena cava, and abdominal aorta

Right and left iliac (inguinal)
■ Include portions of the small and large intestines

Hypogastric (pubic)
■ Contains a portion of the sigmoid colon, urinary bladder and ureters, and portions of the small intestine

Cells

Cells are the body's basic building blocks. They're the smallest living components of an organism. The human body consists of millions of cells grouped into highly specialized units that function together throughout the organism's life. Large groups of individual cells form tissues, such as muscle and blood. In turn, tissues form the organs (such as the brain and heart) that are integrated into body systems (such as the central nervous system [CNS] and cardiovascular system).

Inside scoop

Inside a cell

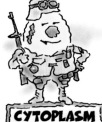

I surround and protect the nucleus.

CYTOPLASM

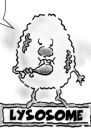

I'm the cell's digestive system.

LYSOSOME

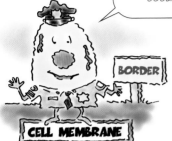

I'm the boundary system for the cell, and I make sure that nothing escapes me!

BORDER

CELL MEMBRANE

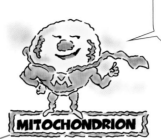

I'm the Mighty Mitochondrion. I give the cell energy.

MITOCHONDRION

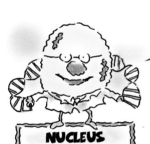

I'm the brain, or control center, of the cell. I carry most of the genetic material, so if you have red hair, it's probably because of me!

NUCLEUS

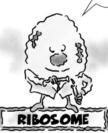

I combine protein and other material the cell needs.

RIBOSOME

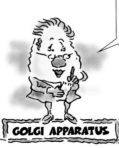

I hold enzyme systems, and I assist in the cell's metabolism.

GOLGI APPARATUS

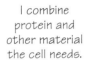

DNA and RNA

Protein synthesis is essential for the growth of new cells and the repair of damaged cells. That's where deoxyribonucleic acid (DNA) and ribonucleic acid (RNA) come into play.

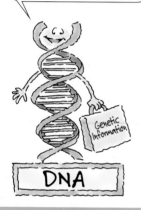

I carry the genetic information that provides the blueprint for protein synthesis.

DNA

■ DNA chains exist in pairs held together by weak chemical attractions between the nitrogen bases on adjacent chains.

■ Because of the chemical shape of the bases, adenine bonds only with thymine and guanine bonds only with cytosine.

■ Bases that can link with each other are called complementary.

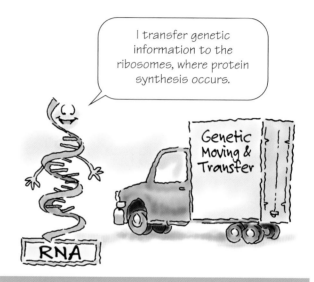

I transfer genetic information to the ribosomes, where protein synthesis occurs.

Genetic Moving & Transfer

RNA

■ RNA consists of nucleotide chains that differ slightly from the nucleotide chains found in DNA.

■ Several types of RNA are involved in the transfer (to the ribosomes) of genetic information essential to protein synthesis.

Types of RNA

Ribosomal RNA

■ Used to make ribosomes in the endoplasmic reticulum of the cytoplasm, where the cell produces proteins

Messenger RNA

■ Directs the arrangement of amino acids to make proteins at the ribosomes

■ Contains a single strand of nucleotides that's complementary to a segment of the DNA chain that contains instructions for protein synthesis

■ Contains chains that pass from the nucleus into the cytoplasm, where they attach to ribosomes

Transfer RNA

■ Consists of short nucleotide chains, each of which is specific for an individual amino acid

■ Transfers the genetic code from messenger RNA for the production of a specific amino acid

Cell reproduction

Cells reproduce through the cell division processes of mitosis and meiosis. Before a cell divides, however, its chromosomes are duplicated. During this process, DNA's double helix separates into two chains.

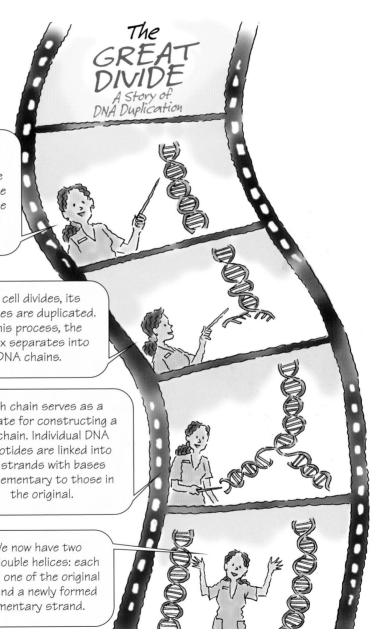

Imagine linked DNA chains as a spiral staircase. The deoxyribose and phosphate groups form the railings; the nitrogen base pairs (adenine and thymine, guanine and cytosine) form the steps.

Before a cell divides, its chromosomes are duplicated. During this process, the double helix separates into two DNA chains.

Each chain serves as a template for constructing a new chain. Individual DNA nucleotides are linked into new strands with bases complementary to those in the original.

This constant pressure to reproduce or die is really starting to take a toll!

Voila! We now have two identical double helices: each containing one of the original strands and a newly formed complementary strand.

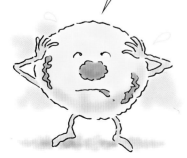

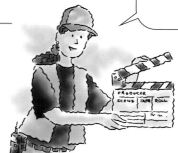

Here's where the action really picks up: the four phases of mitosis.

Mitosis

Mitosis is the equal division of material in the nucleus, followed by division of the cell body. Before division, a cell must double its mass and content. This occurs during the growth phase, called *interphase* (not illustrated). During this phase, chromatin (the small, slender rods of the nucleus that produce its granular appearance) begins to form.

1 Prophase

The chromosomes coil and shorten, and the nuclear membrane dissolves. Each chromosome consists of a pair of strands called *chromatids,* which are connected by a spindle of fibers called a *centromere.*

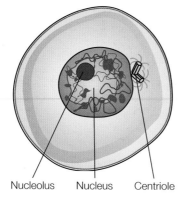

Nucleolus   Nucleus   Centriole

2 Metaphase

The centromeres divide, pulling the chromosomes apart. The centromeres then align themselves in the middle of the spindle.

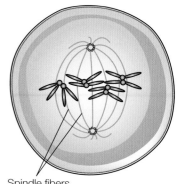

Spindle fibers

3 Anaphase

At the onset of anaphase, the centromeres begin to separate and pull the newly replicated chromosomes toward opposite sides of the cell. By the end of anaphase, 46 chromosomes are present on each side of the cell.

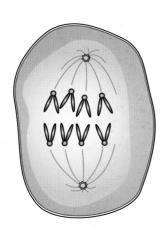

4 Telophase

A new membrane forms around each set of 46 chromosomes. The spindle fibers disappear, cytokinesis occurs, and the cytoplasm divides, producing two new identical daughter cells.

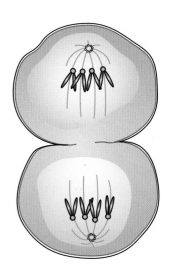

Meiosis

Reserved for gametes (ova and spermatozoa), the process of meiosis intermixes genetic material between homologous chromosomes, producing four daughter cells, each with the haploid number of chromosomes (23, or half of the 46). Meiosis has two divisions separated by a resting phase.

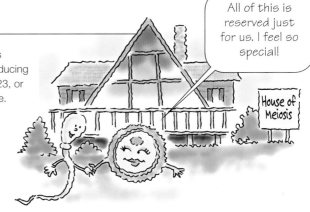

All of this is reserved just for us. I feel so special!

House of Meiosis

1
First division

The first division has six phases. Here's what happens during each.

Interphase

1. Chromosomes replicate, forming a double strand attached at the center by a centromere.
2. Chromosomes appear as an indistinguishable matrix within the nucleus.
3. Centrioles appear outside the nucleus.

Prophase I

1. The nucleolus and nuclear membrane disappear.
2. Chromosomes are distinct, with chromatids attached by the centromere.
3. Homologous chromosomes move close together and inter-twine; exchange of genetic information (genetic recombination) may occur.
4. Centrioles separate, and spindle fibers appear.

Metaphase I

1. Pairs of synaptic chromosomes line up randomly along the metaphase plate.
2. Spindle fibers attach to each chromosome pair.

Anaphase I

1. Synaptic pairs separate.
2. Spindle fibers pull homologous, double-stranded chromosomes to opposite ends of the cell.
3. Chromatids remain attached.

Telophase I

1. The nuclear membrane forms.
2. Spindle fibers and chromosomes disappear.
3. Cytoplasm compresses and divides the cell in half.
4. Each new cell contains the haploid (23) number of chromosomes.

Interkinesis

1. The nucleus and nuclear membrane are well defined.
2. The nucleolus is prominent, and each chromosome has two chromatids that don't replicate.

2
Second division

The second division closely resembles mitosis and is characterized by these four phases.

Prophase II

1. The nuclear membrane disappears.
2. Spindle fibers form.
3. Double-stranded chromosomes appear as thin threads.

Metaphase II

1. Chromosomes line up along the metaphase plate.
2. Centromeres replicate.

Anaphase II

1. Chromatids separate (now a single-stranded chromosome).
2. Chromosomes move away from each other to the opposite ends of the cell.

Telophase II

1. The nuclear membrane forms.
2. Chromosomes and spindle fibers disappear.
3. Cytoplasm compresses, dividing the cell in half.
4. Four daughter cells are created, each of which contains the haploid (23) number of chromosomes.

Movement within cells

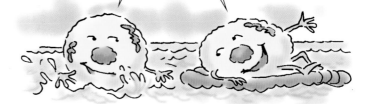

It isn't like we just get to sit around. We're always interacting with body fluids to swap substances.

I like the passive transport mechanisms—such as diffusion and osmosis—the best. They don't require any energy.

Passive transport

Diffusion

In diffusion, solutes move from an area of higher concentration to one of lower concentration. Eventually, an equal distribution of solutes between the two areas occurs.

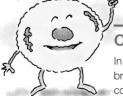

Oh, I get it! In diffusion, the solutes move. In osmosis, the fluid moves. If this is osmosis, my solutes are staying put!

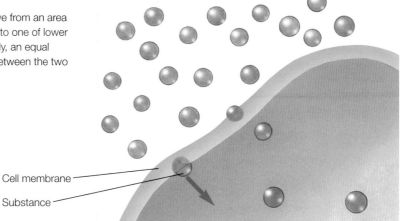

Cell membrane

Substance

Osmosis

In osmosis, fluid moves across a membrane from an area of lower solute concentration (comparatively more fluid) to an area of higher solute concentration (comparatively less fluid). Osmosis stops when enough fluid has moved through the membrane to equalize the solute concentration on both sides of the membrane.

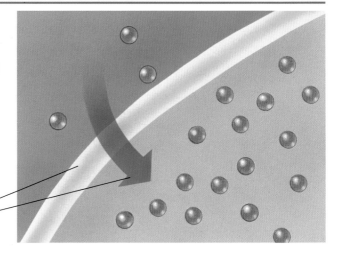

Cell membrane

Fluid

Active transport

Sodium-potassium pump

The sodium-potassium pump moves sodium from inside the cell to outside, where the sodium concentration is greater; potassium moves from outside the cell to inside, where the potassium concentration is greater. Adenosine triphosphate (ATP) provides the energy required for this movement.

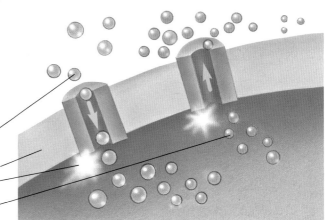

Potassium

Cell membrane

ATP

Sodium

Pinocytosis

In pinocytosis, tiny vacuoles take droplets of fluid containing dissolved substances into the cell. The engulfed fluid is used in the cell.

Vacuole

Cell membrane

Fluid with dissolved substances

Filtration

In filtration, pressure (provided by capillary blood) forces fluid and dissolved particles through the cell membrane and into the interstitial fluid.

The rate of filtration—or how quickly substances pass through the membrane—depends on the amount of pressure.

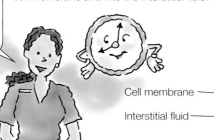

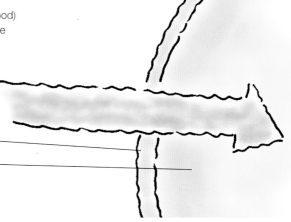

Cell membrane

Interstitial fluid

Tissue

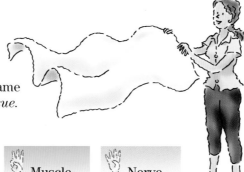

Groups of cells that perform the same general function are known as *tissue*. The body has four types of tissue:

> Epithelial tissue, or epithelium, is a continuous cellular sheet that covers the body's surface, lines body cavities, and forms certain glands.

 Epithelial   Connective   Muscle   Nerve

Epithelial tissue

Epithelial tissue is classified by the number of cell **LAYERS** and the **SHAPE** of surface cells.

Number of cell layers

- *Simple*: One layer
- *Stratified*: Multilayered
- *Pseudostratified*: One layer but appearing to be multilayered

Shape of surface cells

- *Squamous*: Containing flat surface cells
- *Columnar*: Containing tall, cylindrical surface cells
- *Cuboidal*: Containing cube-shaped surface cells

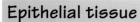 Inside scoop

Types of epithelial tissue

Simple squamous
- Single layer of flattened cells with disc-shaped nuclei
- Lines blood vessels, lymph nodes, and the alveoli of the lungs

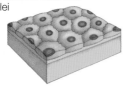

Simple columnar epithelium
- Single layer of tall cells with oval nuclei
- Lines the intestines

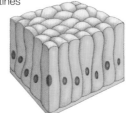

Stratified squamous epithelium
- Basal cells that are cuboidal or columnar
- Makes up the epidermis of the skin

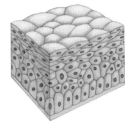

Simple cuboidal epithelium
- Single layer of cubelike cells
- Found on the surface of the ovary and the thyroid

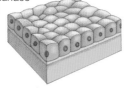

Stratified columnar epithelium
- Superficial cells that are elongated and columnar
- Found in the ducts

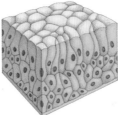

Pseudostratified columnar epithelium
- Cells of different heights with nuclei at different levels
- Form the lining of the respiratory tract (pseudostratified ciliated columnar epithelium with goblet cells)

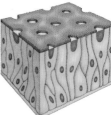

Connective tissue

LOOSE connective tissue

- Contains large spaces that separate the fibers and cells
- Contains a lot of intercellular fluid

DENSE connective tissue

- Provides structural support
- Has greater fiber concentration
- Is subdivided into dense regular and dense irregular connective tissue

Dense regular

- Consists of tightly packed fibers arranged in a consistent pattern
- Includes tendons, ligaments, and aponeuroses (flat fibrous sheets that attach muscles to bones or other tissues)

Dense irregular

- Has tightly packed fibers arranged in an inconsistent pattern
- Found in the dermis, submucosa of the GI tract, fibrous capsules, and fasciae

→ Inside scoop

Adipose tissue

Commonly called *fat*, adipose tissue is a specialized type of loose connective tissue. Widely distributed subcutaneously, adipose tissue acts as insulation to conserve body heat, as a cushion for internal organs, and as a storage depot for excess food and reserve supplies of energy.

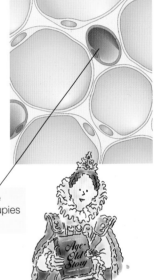

In this tissue, a single lipid (fat) droplet occupies most of each cell.

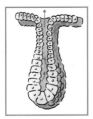

Age-old story

Fat distribution

In men

- Nape of the neck
- Region over seventh cervical vertebra
- Deltoid muscle
- Triceps muscle
- Lumbosacral region
- Buttocks
- Abdomen

In women

- Breasts
- Buttocks
- Thighs
- Abdomen

Glandular epithelium

Organs that produce secretions consist of a special type of epithelium called *glandular epithelium*. Glands are classified as exocrine or endocrine according to how they secrete their products.

- **Endocrine glands** release their secretions into the blood or lymph. (For instance, the medulla of the adrenal gland secretes epinephrine and norepinephrine into the bloodstream.)

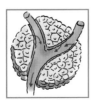

- **Exocrine glands** discharge their secretions onto external or internal surfaces. (For example, sweat glands secrete sweat onto the surface of the skin.)

Mixed glands, such as the pancreas, perform the roles of both endocrine and exocrine glands.

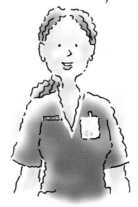

Muscle tissue

Muscle tissue consists of muscle cells with a generous blood supply. Muscle cells measure up to several centimeters long and have an elongated shape that enhances their contractility.

Inside scoop
Types of muscle tissue

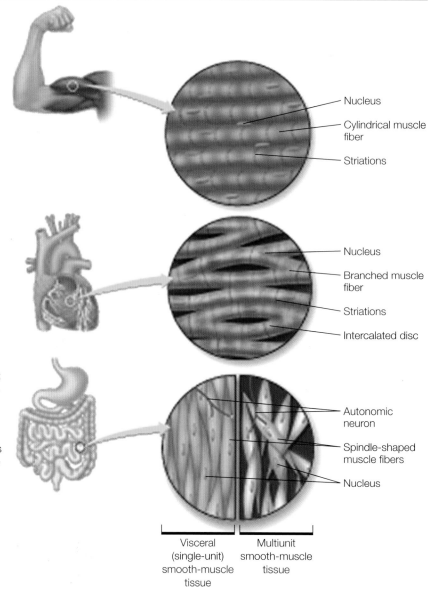

Striated muscle
- Has striped appearance
- Contracts voluntarily
- Found in all muscles that move or stabilize the skeleton: muscles that guard entrances and exits of digestive, respiratory, and urinary tracts

Nucleus

Cylindrical muscle fiber

Striations

Cardiac muscle
- Sometimes classified as striated tissue because of its striped appearance but differs from striated tissue
  – Has fibers that are separate cellular units without many nuclei
  – Contracts involuntarily
  – Found in the heart

Nucleus

Branched muscle fiber

Striations

Intercalated disc

Smooth muscle
- Consists of long, spindle-shaped cells; lacks the striped pattern of striated tissue
- Stimulated by the autonomic nervous system
- Isn't under voluntary control
- Lines the walls of many internal organs and other structures, including respiratory passages, urinary and genital ducts, arteries and veins, larger lymphatic trunks, arrectores pilorum (tiny muscles that act as the hair erector muscles), and the iris and ciliary body of the eyes

Autonomic neuron

Spindle-shaped muscle fibers

Nucleus

Visceral (single-unit) smooth-muscle tissue

Multiunit smooth-muscle tissue

Nerve tissue

Neurons are highly specialized cells composed of nerve tissue that generates and conducts nerve impulses. Its primary properties are:

IRRITABILITY : the capacity to react to various physical and chemical agents, and

CONDUCTIVITY : the ability to transmit the resulting reaction from one point to another.

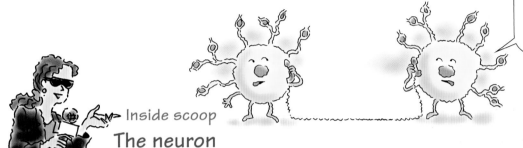

Can you hear me now? After all, the main function of nerve tissue is communication.

→ Inside scoop

The neuron

A typical neuron consists of a cell body with cytoplasmic extensions—numerous dendrites on one pole and a single axon on the opposite pole. These extensions allow the neuron to conduct impulses over long distances.

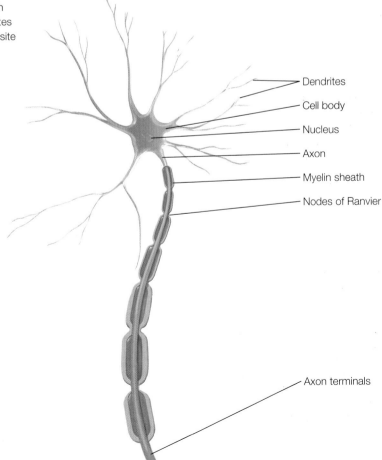

Dendrites

Cell body

Nucleus

Axon

Myelin sheath

Nodes of Ranvier

Axon terminals

VISION QUEST

Able to label?

Identify the abdominal regions shown on this illustration.

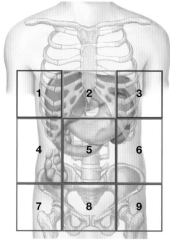

1. _____
2. _____
3. _____
4. _____
5. _____
8. _____
7. _____
8. _____
9. _____

Matchmaker

Match the four forms of movement within cells illustrated here with their definitions.

1. _____

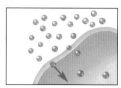

2. _____

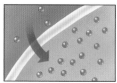

3. _____

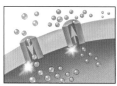

4. _____

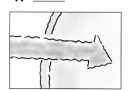

A. Movement of sodium from inside the cell to outside, where sodium concentration is greater, and movement of potassium from outside the cell to inside, where potassium concentration is greater

B. Passive movement of fluid across a membrane, from an area of lower solute concentration into an area of higher solute concentration

C. Passive movement of solutes from an area of higher concentration to an area of lower concentration

D. Movement of fluid and dissolved particles through a cell membrane as a result of pressure on one side of the membrane

Answers: Able to label? 1. Right hypochondriac, 2. Epigastric, 3. Left hypochondriac, 4. Right lumbar (lateral), 5. Umbilical, 6. Left lumbar (lateral), 7. Right iliac (inguinal), 8. Hypogastric, 9. Left iliac (inguinal); Matchmaker 1. C (diffusion), 2. B (osmosis), 3. A (sodium-potassium pump), 4. D (filtration).

2 Genetics

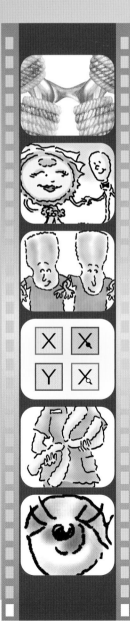

- Genetics basics 20
- Genes 21
- Vision quest 24

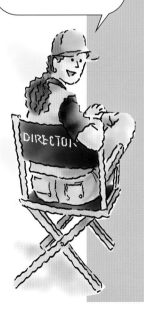

Sometimes the real story goes on behind the camera. Sort of like genes…you may not see them, but they know how to exert their influence.

DIRECTOR

Genetics basics

Genetics is the study of heredity—the passing of traits from biological parents to their children. Physical traits, such as eye color, are inherited, as are biochemical and physiologic traits, including the tendency to develop certain diseases.

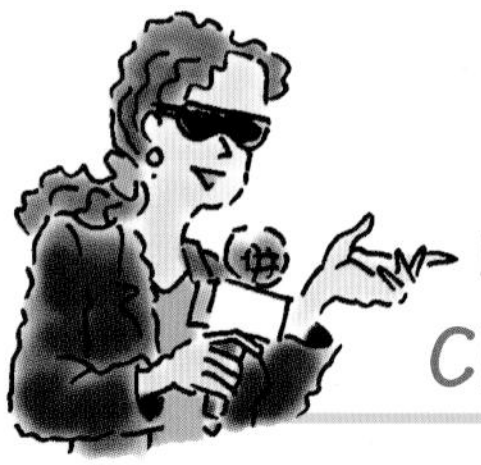

Inside scoop

Chromosomes

A chromosome is made up of deoxyribonucleic acid (DNA) molecules coiled around a protein framework.

Centromere

DNA coiled around a protein framework

Protein framework

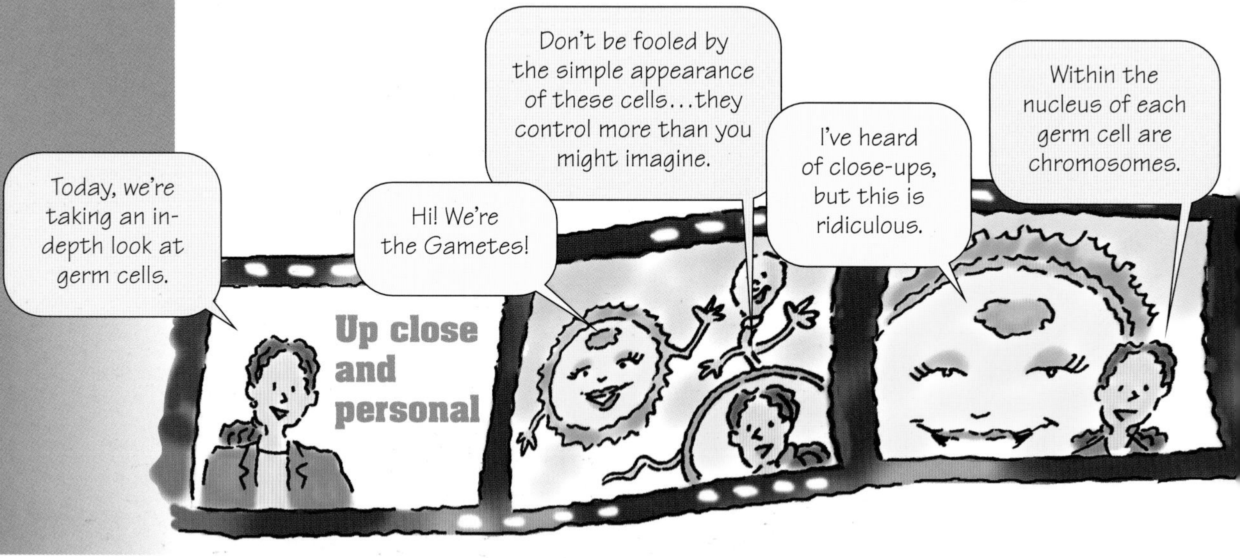

Today, we're taking an in-depth look at germ cells.

Hi! We're the Gametes!

Don't be fooled by the simple appearance of these cells...they control more than you might imagine.

I've heard of close-ups, but this is ridiculous.

Within the nucleus of each germ cell are chromosomes.

Up close and personal

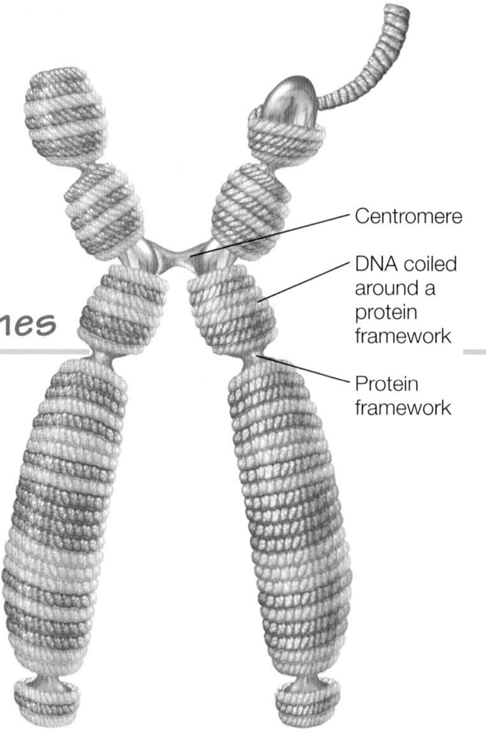

Genes

Genes are segments of chromosomal DNA chains that are responsible for inherited traits. Each parent contributes one set of chromosomes (and therefore one set of genes) so that every offspring has two genes for every location on the autosomal chromosomes.

Variations in a particular gene—such as brown, blue, or green eye color—are called *alleles*. The effect that gene has on cell structure or function is called *gene expression*. Gene expression can vary with the gene.

 Normal cells contain 23 pairs of chromosomes

 22 pairs are sets of chromosomes that contain genetic information

 1 pair is composed of sex (X and Y) chromosomes

 The composition of the X and Y chromosomes determines sex
– XY is genetically male
– XX is genetically female

How genes express themselves

Dominant genes

If genes could speak, dominant genes would be loud and garrulous, dominating every conversation! Dominant genes (such as the one for dark hair) can be expressed and transmitted to the offspring even if only one parent possesses the gene.

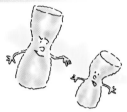

Recessive genes

Unlike dominant genes, recessive genes prefer to hide their light under a bushel basket. A recessive gene (such as the one for blond hair) is expressed only when both parents transmit it to the offspring.

Codominant genes

Firm believers in equality, codominant genes (such as the genes that direct specific types of hemoglobin synthesis in red blood cells) allow expression of both alleles.

Sex-linked genes

Sex-linked genes are carried on sex chromosomes. Almost all appear on the X chromosome and are recessive. In the male, sex-linked genes behave like dominant genes because no second X chromosome exists.

> That's a man for you. Who else would interpret a lack of genetic material as an asset?

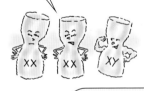

> Each chromosome contains a strand of DNA.

> Along the strand of DNA are thousands of genes.

> Each gene carries the traits that a person inherits, including everything from blood type to toe shape.

> When these seemingly simple cells unite at fertilization, they determine a person's entire genetic inheritance.

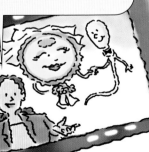

Understanding autosomal dominant inheritance

This diagram shows the possible offspring of a parent with recessive normal genes (aa) and a parent with an altered dominant gene (Aa). *Note:* With each pregnancy, the offspring has a 50% chance of being affected.

A dominant gene is expressed even if only one parent transmits it to the offspring. Dark hair can result from dominant genes.

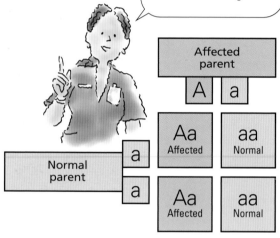

Understanding autosomal recessive inheritance

This diagram shows the possible offspring of two unaffected parents, each with an altered recessive gene (a) on an autosome. Each offspring will have a one-in-four chance of being affected and a two-in-four chance of being a carrier.

A recessive gene is expressed only when both parents transmit it to the offspring. Blond hair and blue eyes result from recessive genes.

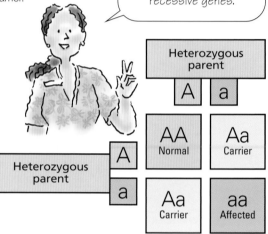

Multifactorial inheritance

Multifactorial inheritance reflects the interaction of at least two abnormal genes and environmental factors. Height is a classic example of a multifactorial trait. In general, the height of offspring will be in a range between the height of the two parents. But nutritional patterns, health care, and other environmental factors also influence development.

Factors contributing to multifactorial inheritance

- Maternal age
- Use of drugs, alcohol, or hormones by either parent
- Maternal or paternal exposure to radiation
- Maternal infection during pregnancy or existing diseases in the mother
- Nutritional factors
- General maternal or paternal health
- High altitude
- Maternal smoking
- Maternal-fetal blood incompatibility
- Inadequate prenatal care

Understanding X-linked dominant inheritance

This diagram shows the possible offspring of a normal parent and a parent with an X-linked dominant gene on the X chromosome (shown by a solid dot). When the father is affected, only his daughters have the abnormal gene. When the mother is affected, both male and female offspring may be affected.

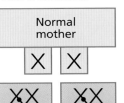

Normal mother

X X

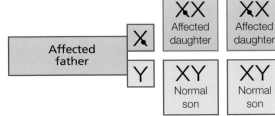

Affected father

X̣ — | X̣X Affected daughter | X̣X Affected daughter |

Y — | XY Normal son | XY Normal son |

Affected mother

X̣ X

Normal father

X — | X̣X Affected daughter | XX Normal daughter |

Y — | X̣Y Affected son | XY Normal son |

Understanding X-linked recessive inheritance

This diagram shows the possible offspring of a normal parent and a parent with a recessive gene on the X chromosome (shown by an open dot). All of the female offspring of an affected male will be carriers. The son of a female carrier may inherit a recessive gene on the X chromosome and be affected by the disease.

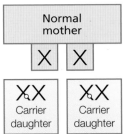

Normal mother

X X

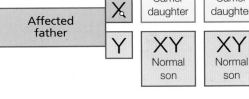

Affected father

X̧ — | X̧X Carrier daughter | X̧X Carrier daughter |

Y — | XY Normal son | XY Normal son |

Carrier mother

X̧ X

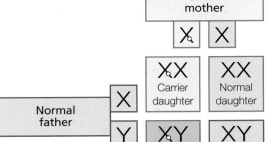

Normal father

X — | X̧X Carrier daughter | XX Normal daughter |

Y — | X̧Y Affected son | XY Normal son |

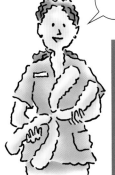

> Sex-linked genes are carried on sex chromosomes. Almost all appear on the X chromosome and are recessive.

X marks the spot

In a male, sex-linked genes behave like dominant genes because males have no second X chromosome. Red-green color-blindness is a result of a recessive X-linked inheritance. Male children of a parent who carries the recessive trait may be color-blind.

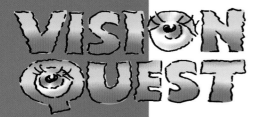

My word!

Use the clues to help you unscramble terms related to genetics. Then use the circled letters to answer the question posed.

Question: Which type of genes allow expression of both alleles?

1. Variations in a particular gene

   leasell

   ◯ — — — — — —

2. Effect a gene has on cell structure or function

   neeg sirensexpo

   — — ◯ —   — — — — — — — — ◯◯

3. Gene that can be expressed and transmitted to offspring even when only one parent possesses it

   nomadtin

   ◯◯◯ — — — — ◯

4. Gene that can be expressed only when both parents transmit it

   iceserves

   — — ◯ — — — ◯ — —

Answer: _ _ _ _ _ _ _ _ _ _

Rebus riddle

Sound out each group of pictures and symbols to reveal a fact about genetics.

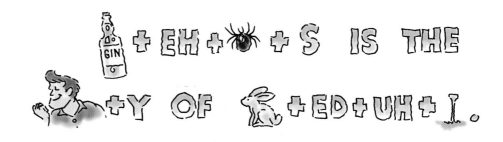

3
Chemical organization

■ The body's chemistry 26

■ Atomic structure 27

■ Inorganic and organic compounds 31

■ Vision quest 34

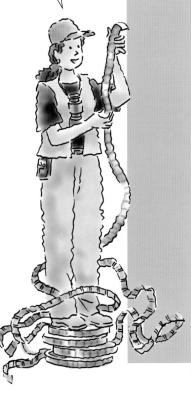

Film is made of celluloid. The body is made of chemicals. Man, nothing is as it seems!

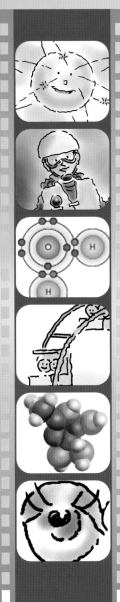

The body's chemistry

All of the body's activities are chemical in nature, making knowledge of chemistry key to understanding the human body and its functions.

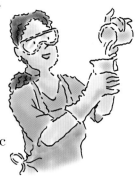

Every cell contains thousands of different chemicals that constantly interact with one another. Differences in chemical composition differentiate types of body tissue. What's more, the blueprints of heredity—deoxyribonucleic acid (DNA) and ribonucleic acid (RNA)—are encoded in chemical form.

	Matter	Energy
	Matter is anything that has mass and occupies space.	Energy is the capacity to do work—to put matter into motion. Energy may be stored (potential energy) or in motion (kinetic energy).
Solid	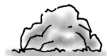	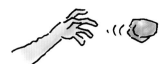
Liquid		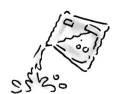
Gas	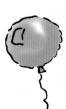	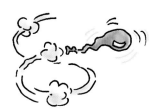

Atomic structure

Understanding the atomic structure starts with knowing the difference between atoms, molecules, and compounds.

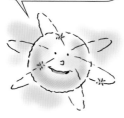

Because I'm a single atom, I can't be broken down. That makes me an element.

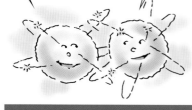

We're atoms that are joined together to make a molecule.

We're the same, so we're a molecule of an element.

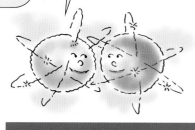

I know we're different. That's why we'll make a beautiful compound.

Atom
■ Smallest unit of matter that can take part in a chemical reaction

Molecule
■ A combination of two or more atoms of the same element (such as hydrogen)

Compound
■ A combination of two or more atoms that are different—that is, different elements (such as a carbon atom and an oxygen atom)

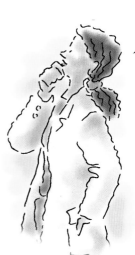

Okay, I think I have it. An element can either be an atom or a molecule, as long as the atoms are all the same.

Subatomic particles

Atoms consist of three basic subatomic particles.

Protons

✚ Protons have a positive charge.
✚ Each element has a distinct number of protons.

Neutrons

■ Neutrons carry a neutral charge.
■ Not all the atoms of an element necessarily have the same number of neutrons.
■ Forms of an atom with a different number of neutrons (and a different atomic weight) than most atoms of the element are called *isotopes*.

Electrons

▬ Electrons carry a negative charge.
▬ Electrons play a key role in chemical bonds and reactions.
▬ The number of electrons in an atom equals the number of protons in its nucleus.
▬ Each electron shell can hold a maximum number of electrons and represents a specific energy level.

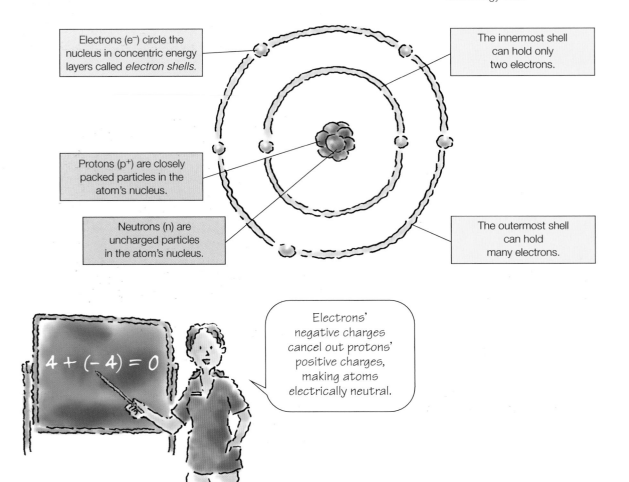

Electrons (e⁻) circle the nucleus in concentric energy layers called *electron shells*.

The innermost shell can hold only two electrons.

Protons (p⁺) are closely packed particles in the atom's nucleus.

Neutrons (n) are uncharged particles in the atom's nucleus.

The outermost shell can hold many electrons.

$$4 + (-4) = 0$$

Electrons' negative charges cancel out protons' positive charges, making atoms electrically neutral.

Chemical reactions

Chemical reactions depend on energy as well as particle concentration, speed, and orientation. A chemical reaction involves unpaired electrons in the outer shells of atoms. In this reaction, one of two events occurs:

Unpaired electrons from the outer shell of one atom transfer to the outer shell of another atom

One atom shares its unpaired electrons with another atom.

Four basic types of chemical reactions

■ **Synthesis:** Two or more substances combine to form a new, more complex substance
$$A + B \rightarrow A B$$

■ **Decomposition:** One substance breaks down into two or more simpler substances
$$A B \rightarrow A + B$$

■ **Exchange:** A combination of decomposition and synthesis
$$A B + C D \rightarrow A + B + C + D \rightarrow A D + B C$$

■ **Reversible:** The product may revert back to its original reactant or vice versa
$$A + B \longleftrightarrow A B$$

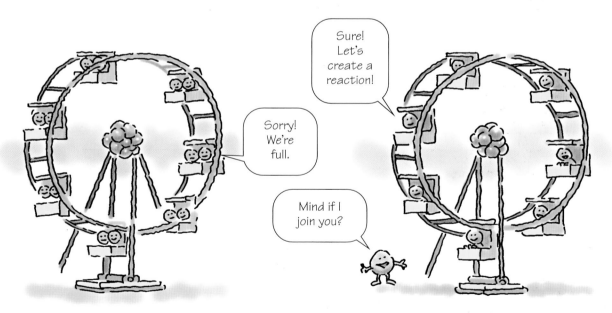

Sure! Let's create a reaction!

Sorry! We're full.

Mind if I join you?

An atom with an outer shell that contains only pairs of electrons is chemically inactive, or stable.

An atom with single (unpaired) electrons orbiting in its outermost electron shell can be chemically active—that is, able to take part in chemical reactions.

Chemical bonds

A chemical bond is a force of attraction that binds a molecule's atoms together.

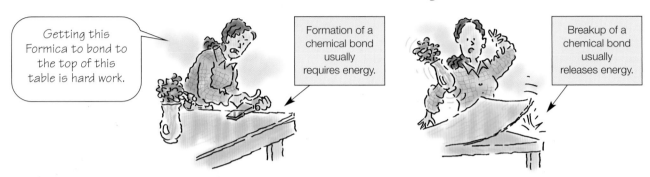

Getting this Formica to bond to the top of this table is hard work.

Formation of a chemical bond usually requires energy.

Breakup of a chemical bond usually releases energy.

Types of chemical bonds

Hydrogen bond

A hydrogen bond occurs when there's an attractive force between the hydrogen attached to an electronegative atom of one molecule and an electronegative atom of another molecule. For example, water molecules are held together by hydrogen bonds.

Oxygen atom (O)

Hydrogen atoms (H)

Water molecule (H_2O)

Hydrogen bonds

Ionic bond

An ionic bond occurs when an electron is transferred from one atom to another. For example, by forces of attraction, an electron is transferred from a sodium (Na) atom to a chlorine (Cl) atom. The result is a molecule of sodium chloride (NaCl).

Sodium atom (Na)

Chlorine atom (Cl)

Sodium ion (Na^+)

Chlorine ion (Cl^-)

Sodium chloride (NaCl)

Covalent bond

In a covalent bond, atoms share a pair of electrons. This is what happens when two hydrogen (H) atoms form a covalent bond.

Hydrogen atom (H)

Hydrogen atom (H)

Hydrogen molecule (H_2)

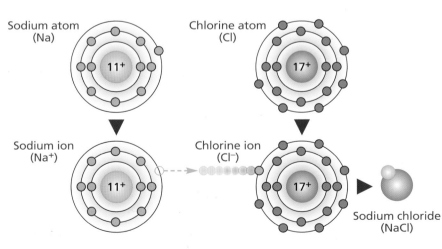

Inorganic and organic compounds

Although most biomolecules (molecules produced by living cells) form *organic compounds*, or compounds containing carbon, some form *inorganic compounds*, or compounds without carbon.

Inorganic compounds

Inorganic compounds are usually small. Examples include water and electrolytes.

Water
- The body's most abundant substance
- Easily forms polar covalent bonds (which permit the transport of solvents)
- Acts as a lubricant in mucus and other bodily fluids
- Enters into chemical reactions (such as nutrient breakdown during digestion)
- Enables the body to maintain a relatively constant temperature

Body fluids must attain acid-base balance to maintain homeostasis (the dynamic equilibrium of the body).

Electrolytes
- Compounds whose molecules consist of positively charged ions, *cations*, and negatively charged ions, *anions*, that separate into ions (*ionize*) in solution
- Include acids, bases, and salts

A solution's acidity is determined by the number of hydrogen ions it contains. The more hydrogen ions present, the more acidic the solution. Conversely, the fewer hydroxide ions a solution contains, the more basic, or alkaline, it is.

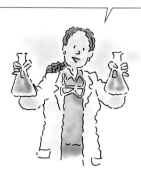

 ionize into hydrogen ions and anions.

 ionize into hydroxide ions and cations.

 form when acids react with bases. In water, they ionize into cations and anions.

Organic compounds

Most biomolecules form *organic compounds*—compounds that contain carbon or carbon-hydrogen bonds. Carbohydrates, lipids, proteins, and nucleic acids are all examples of organic compounds.

Carbohydrates

In the body, carbohydrates are sugars, starches, glycogen, and cellulose.
There are three types of carbohydrates:

Carbohydrate molecule

Monosaccharides, such as ribose and deoxyribose, are sugars with three to seven carbon atoms.

Disaccharides, such as lactose and maltose, contain two monosaccharides.

Polysaccharides, such as glycogen, are large carbohydrates with many monosaccharides.

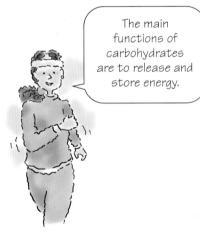

The main functions of carbohydrates are to release and store energy.

Lipids

Lipids are water-insoluble biomolecules. The major lipids are:

Lipid molecule

Triglycerides
- Most abundant lipids in both food and the body
- Neutral fats that insulate and protect
- The body's most concentrated energy source

Lipoproteins
- Help transport lipids to various parts of the body

Sterols
- Simple lipids with no fatty acids in their molecules
- Fall into four main categories:

  Bile salts: emulsify fats during digestion and aid absorption of the fat-soluble vitamins (vitamins A, D, E, and K)

  Male and female sex hormones: responsible for sexual characteristics and reproduction

  Cholesterol: a part of animal cell membranes; needed to form all other sterols

  Vitamin D: helps regulate the body's calcium concentration

Phospholipids
- Major structural components of cell membranes
- Consist of one molecule of glycerol, two molecules of a fatty acid, and a phosphate group

Eicosanoids
- Prostaglandins: modify hormone responses, promote the inflammatory response, and open the airways
- Leukotrienes: play a part in allergic and inflammatory responses

Proteins

Proteins are the most abundant organic compound in the body. Many amino acids linked together form a polypeptide. One or more polypeptides form a protein.

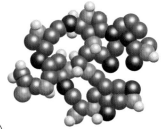

Protein molecule

> Proteins are composed of amino acid building blocks linked together by peptide bonds.

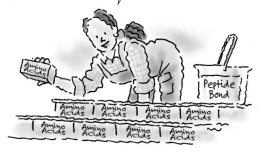

A protein's shape determines which function it performs:
- providing structure and protection
- promoting muscle contraction
- transporting various substances
- regulating processes
- serving as enzymes (the largest group of proteins, which act as catalysts for crucial chemical reactions).

Nucleic acids

The nucleic acids DNA and RNA are composed of nitrogenous bases, sugars, and phosphate groups.

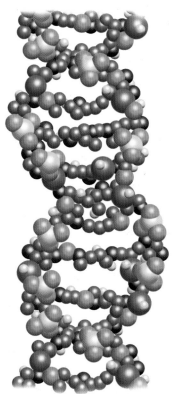

Nucleic acid

> The primary hereditary molecule, DNA contains two long chains of deoxyribonucleotides, which coil into a double-helix shape.

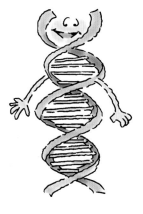

VISION QUEST

Able to label?

Identify the parts of the atom shown in this illustration.

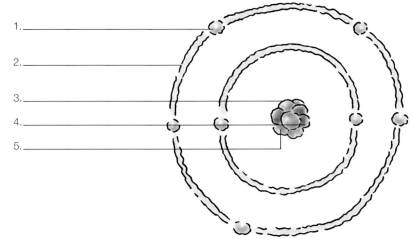

1. _____
2. _____
3. _____
4. _____
5. _____

My word!

Use the clues to help you unscramble terms related to the body's chemistry. Then use the circled letters to answer the question posed.

Question: What's the most abundant organic compound in the body?

1. Term used to describe something that has mass and occupies space

   artmet   _ _ ⃝ _ ⃝⃝

2. Smallest unit of matter that can take part in a chemical reaction

   moat   _ _ ⃝ _

3. Term that describes a combination of two or more atoms that are different

   copmudno   _ _ _ ⃝ _ _ ⃝ _

4. An atom with a different number of neutrons than usual

   piestoo   ⃝ _ _ _ _ _ _

Answer: _ _ _ _ _ _ _

4 Integumentary system

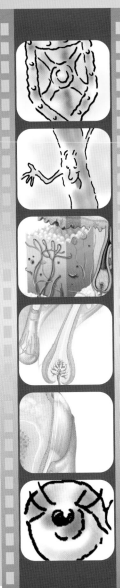

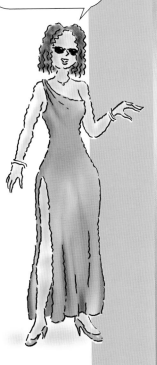

People may think I'm shallow for caring so much about my skin, but I know about all the activity that goes on "behind the scenes."

Skin layers 36

Skin functions 38

Epidermal appendages 40

Vision quest 42

Skin layers

Two distinct layers of skin, the epidermis and dermis, lie above a
third layer of subcutaneous tissue—sometimes called the *hypodermis*.

Inside scoop
Cross-section
of the skin

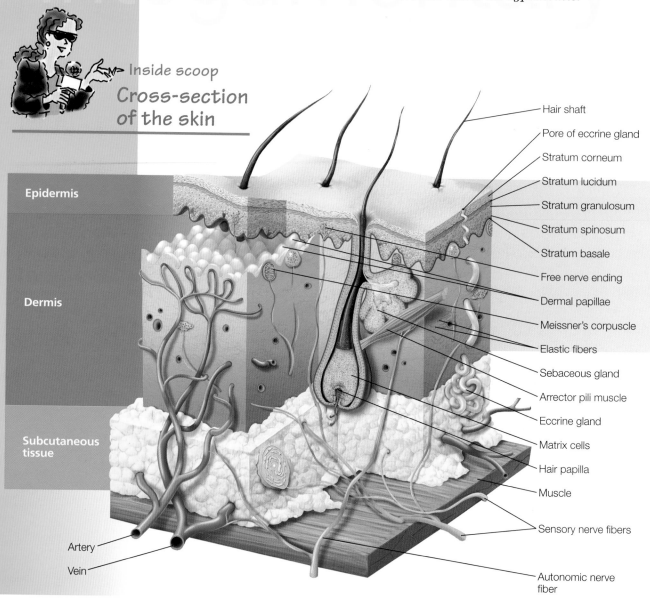

Epidermis

Dermis

Subcutaneous
tissue

Hair shaft

Pore of eccrine gland

Stratum corneum

Stratum lucidum

Stratum granulosum

Stratum spinosum

Stratum basale

Free nerve ending

Dermal papillae

Meissner's corpuscle

Elastic fibers

Sebaceous gland

Arrector pili muscle

Eccrine gland

Matrix cells

Hair papilla

Muscle

Sensory nerve fibers

Autonomic nerve
fiber

Artery

Vein

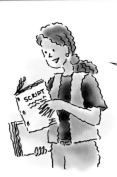

I love a complex plot. The story of the skin involves multiple layers, all working together.

Layer	Sublayers
Epidermis ▪ Outermost layer ▪ Varies in thickness from less than 0.1 mm (on the eyelids) to more than 1 mm (on the palms and soles) ▪ Composed of avascular, stratified, squamous (scaly or platelike) epithelial tissue ▪ Consists of five sublayers	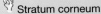 Stratum corneum ▪ Outermost layer ▪ Consists of tightly arranged layers of cellular membranes and keratin Stratum lucidum ▪ Lucid or clear layer ▪ Blocks water penetration or loss Stratum granulosum ▪ Granular layer ▪ Responsible for keratin formation Stratum spinosum ▪ Spiny layer ▪ Helps with keratin formation ▪ Contains a rich supply of ribonucleic acid Stratum basale (basal layer) ▪ Innermost layer ▪ Produces new cells to replace superficial keratinized cells that are continuously shed or worn away
Dermis ▪ Also called the *corium* ▪ Contains and supports blood vessels, lymphatic vessels, nerves, and the epidermal appendages ▪ Composed primarily of matrix, which contains collagen (gives strength), elastin (provides elasticity), and reticular fibers (bind collagen and elastin fibers together) ▪ Consists of two sublayers	 Papillary dermis ▪ Contains fingerlike projections (papillae) that connect the dermis to the epidermis ▪ Contains characteristic ridges Reticular dermis ▪ Covers a layer of subcutaneous tissue, insulating the body to conserve heat ▪ Provides energy ▪ Serves as a mechanical shock absorber

The characteristic ridges of the papillary dermis create fingerprints. They also come in handy by helping the fingers and toes grip surfaces.

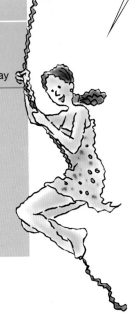

Skin functions

The integumentary system is the largest body system. In addition to the skin, or integument, it includes the hair, nails, and certain glands.

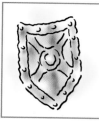

Protection

■ Maintains the integrity of the body surface (through skin migration and shedding)
■ Repairs surface wounds (by intensifying normal cell replacement)
■ Protects the body against noxious chemicals and invasion from bacteria and microorganisms
■ Contains Langerhans' cells (specialized cells in the skin's top layer) that enhance the body's immune response
■ Contains melanocytes (which produce the brown pigment melanin) that help filter ultraviolet light

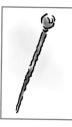

Sensory perception

■ Contains sensory nerve fibers that supply specific areas of the skin (dermatomes)
■ Allows for perception of temperature, touch, pressure, pain, and itching
■ Contains autonomic nerve fibers that carry impulses to smooth muscle in the walls of the skin's blood vessels, to the muscles around the hair roots, and to the sweat glands

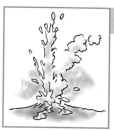

Excretion

■ Excretes sweat, which contains water, electrolytes, urea, and lactic acid
■ Prevents dehydration by regulating the content and volume of sweat
■ Prevents unwanted fluids in the environment from entering the body

It's hard to believe that something as thin as the skin can perform so many functions.

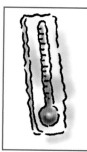

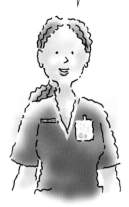

Body temperature

■ Contains nerves, blood vessels, and eccrine glands within the skin's deeper layer to control body temperature
■ Causes blood vessels to constrict (reducing blood flow and conserving heat) when exposed to cold or internal body temperature falls
■ Causes small arteries within the skin to dilate (increasing the blood flow and reducing body heat) when skin becomes too hot or internal body temperature rises

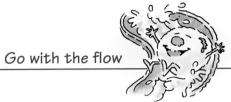

Go with the flow

The skin's role in thermoregulation

Abundant nerves, blood vessels, and eccrine glands within the skin's deeper layer aid thermoregulation (control of body temperature). The first part of the flow chart shows how the body conserves body heat. The second part of the flow chart shows how the body reduces body heat. Here's how the skin does its job.

Time to warm up

1

The skin becomes exposed to cold, or internal body temperature falls.

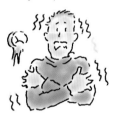

2

Blood vessels constrict in response to stimuli from the autonomic nervous system.

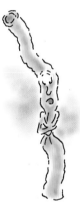

3

Blood flow decreases through the skin, and body heat is conserved.

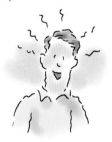

Now let's cool things off

6

Increased blood flow reduces body heat. If this doesn't lower temperature, the eccrine glands act to increase sweat production, and evaporation cools the skin.

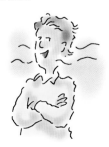

5

Small arteries in the second skin layer (dermis) dilate (expand).

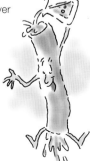

4

The skin becomes too hot, or internal body temperature rises.

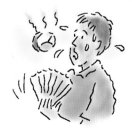

Epidermal appendages

Numerous epidermal appendages occur throughout the skin. They include the hair, nails, sebaceous glands, and sweat glands.

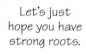

It's hard to believe that hairs are really long, slender shafts composed of keratin.

Let's just hope you have strong roots.

Hair

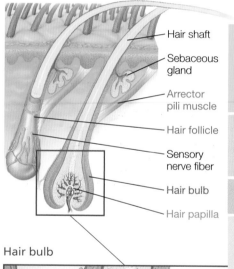

- Hair shaft
- Sebaceous gland
- Arrector pili muscle
- Hair follicle
- Sensory nerve fiber
- Hair bulb
- Hair papilla

Arrector pili, a bundle of smooth-muscle fibers, extend through the dermis to attach to the base of the follicle. When these muscles contract, the hair stands on end.

Each hair lies within an epithelium-lined sheath called a **hair follicle**. Hair follicles have a rich blood and nerve supply.

At the expanded lower end of each hair is a **bulb** or **root**.

On its undersurface, the root is indented by a **hair papilla,** a cluster of connective tissue and blood vessels that provide nourishment to the hair.

Hair bulb

- Matrix cell
  - Produces hair
- Cuticle cells
- Inner root sheath
- Outer root sheath
- Capillary in hair papilla
- Melanocyte
  - Determines hair color

Nails

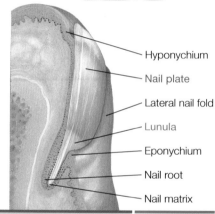

- Hyponychium
- Nail plate
- Lateral nail fold
- Lunula
- Eponychium
- Nail root
- Nail matrix

The **nail plate** (surrounded on three sides by the nail folds, or cuticles) lies on the nail bed. It's formed by the nail matrix, which extends proximally for about ¼″ (0.6 cm) beneath the nail fold. The vascular bed imparts the characteristic pink appearance under the nails.

The **lunula** is where the distal portion of the matrix shows through as a pale, crescent moon–shaped area.

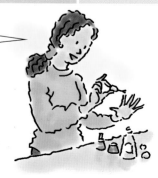

And nails are more than just something to polish. They're also specialized types of keratin.

Sebaceous glands

Sebaceous glands occur on all parts of the skin—except the palms and soles. However, they're most prominent on the scalp, face, upper torso, and genitalia.

| Sebaceous glands produce sebum (a mixture of keratin, fat, and cellulose debris). | → | Sebum combines with sweat to form a moist, oily, acidic film that's mildly antibacterial and antifungal and that protects the skin surface. | → | Sebum exits through the hair follicle opening to reach the skin surface. |

Sweat glands

There are two types of sweat glands.

Eccrine glands

- Widely distributed throughout the body
- Produce an odorless, watery fluid with a sodium concentration equal to that of plasma
- Each contains a duct that passes from the coiled secretory portion, through the dermis and epidermis, and onto the skin surface
- Secrete fluid in response to emotional stress (glands in palms and soles) or thermal stress (to regulate body temperature)

Apocrine glands

- Located chiefly in the axillary (underarm) and anogenital (groin) areas
- Lie deeper in the dermis than eccrine glands
- Each contains a duct that connects the coiled secretory portion to the upper portion of the hair follicle
- Begin to function at puberty
- Have no known biological function
- Bacteria decompose fluids produced by these glands, resulting in body odor

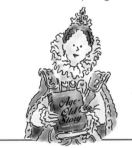

Age-old story

Integumentary timeline

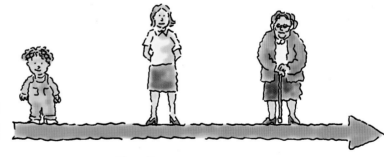

Changes	Results
Loss of subcutaneous fat, thinning dermis, decreased collagen and elastin, decline in cell replacement	Lines around eyes (crow's feet), mouth, and nose
Decreased rate of skin cell replacement	Slowed wound healing with tendency toward infection
Decreased sweat gland output and number of active sweat glands	Dry mucous membranes
Loss of subcutaneous fat (combined with decreased size, number, and function of sweat glands)	Difficulty regulating body temperature
Decreased melanocyte production along with localized proliferation of melanocytes	Development of brown spots (senile lentigo)
Decreased hair pigment	Thinning and graying of hair

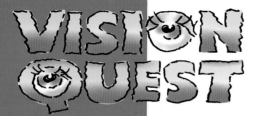

My word!

Unscramble the words using the clues provided. Then use the circled letters to answer the question posed.

Question: Which sweat glands secrete an odorless fluid in response to emotional or thermal stress?

1. **Skin layer that contains blood vessels**

   ridsme _ _ ⊙ _ _ _

2. **Outermost layer of the skin**

   impedesir _ _ _ _ _ ⊙ _ _ ⊙ _

3. **Cells that produce a brown pigment to help filter ultraviolet light**

   castlemoney _ _ _ _ _ ⊙ _ ⊙ _ _ _ _

4. **Smooth-muscle fibers that make hair "stand on end" when they contract**

   carrotre lipi _ _ _ ⊙⊙ _ _ _   _ _ _ _

Answer: _ _ _ _ _ _ _ _

Able to label?

Identify the hair structures shown in the illustration.

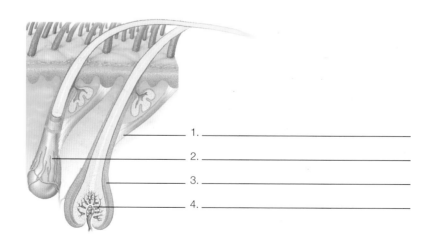

1. _____
2. _____
3. _____
4. _____

Answers: My word! 1. Dermis, 2. Epidermis, 3. Melanocytes, 4. Arrector pili; Question: Eccrine; Able to label? 1. Arrector pili muscle, 2. Hair follicle, 3. Hair bulb, 4. Hair papilla.

5 Musculoskeletal system

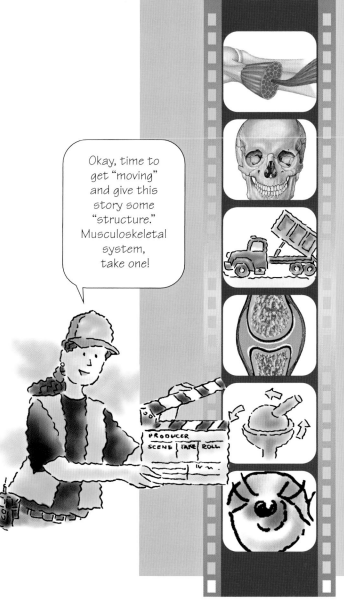

- Muscles 44
- Tendons and ligaments 49
- Bones 50
- Cartilage 54
- Joints 54
- Bursae 55
- Vision quest 56

Okay, time to get "moving" and give this story some "structure." Musculoskeletal system, take one!

Muscles

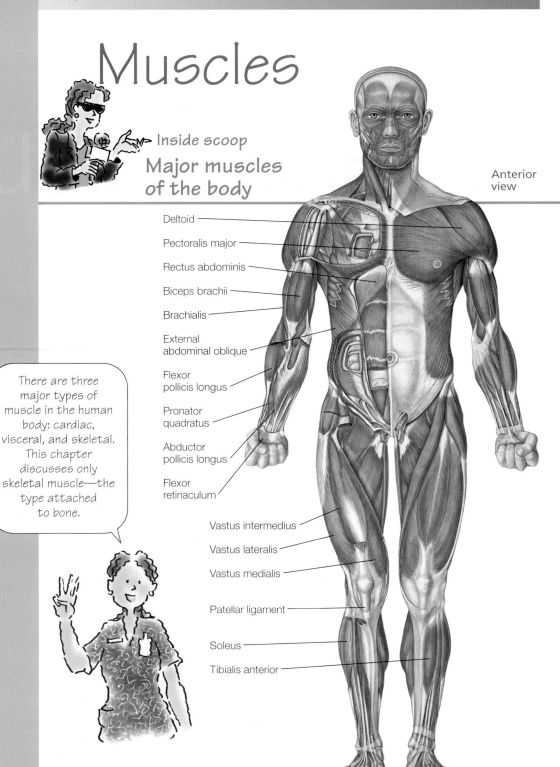

Inside scoop

Major muscles of the body

Anterior view

Deltoid
Pectoralis major
Rectus abdominis
Biceps brachii
Brachialis
External abdominal oblique
Flexor pollicis longus
Pronator quadratus
Abductor pollicis longus
Flexor retinaculum
Vastus intermedius
Vastus lateralis
Vastus medialis
Patellar ligament
Soleus
Tibialis anterior

There are three major types of muscle in the human body: cardiac, visceral, and skeletal. This chapter discusses only skeletal muscle—the type attached to bone.

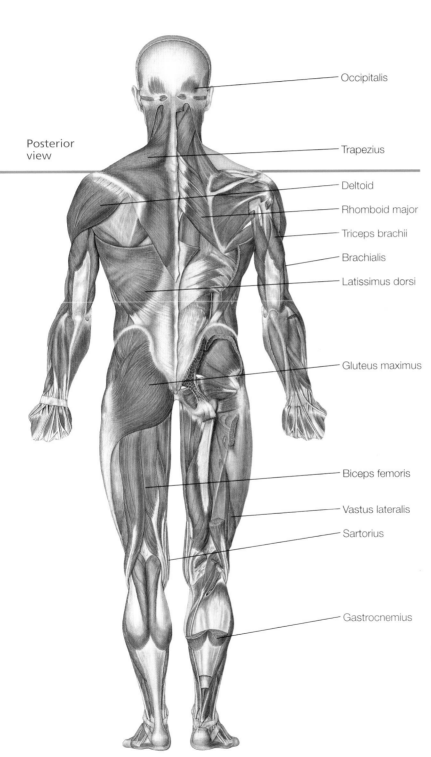

Posterior view

Occipitalis

Trapezius

Deltoid

Rhomboid major

Triceps brachii

Brachialis

Latissimus dorsi

Gluteus maximus

Biceps femoris

Vastus lateralis

Sartorius

Gastrocnemius

Muscles of the axial skeleton

The muscles of the axial skeleton are essential for respiration. The axial skeleton includes:
- muscles of the face, tongue, and neck
- muscles of mastication
- muscles of the vertebral column situated along the spine.

Muscles of the appendicular skeleton

The appendicular skeleton includes the muscles of the:
- shoulder
- abdominopelvic cavity
- upper and lower extremities.

Muscles of the upper extremities are classified according to the bones they move. Those that move the arm are further categorized into those with an origin on the axial skeleton and those with an origin on the scapula.

To remember the muscles of the axial skeleton, think about the muscles along my central line, or axis. To recall the muscles of the appendicular skeleton, think about the muscles related to my appendages, or arms and legs.

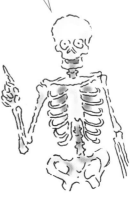

Muscle structure

Skeletal muscle is composed of large, long cell groups called *muscle fibers*. Each fiber has many nuclei and a series of increasingly smaller internal fibrous structures.

Let's move in for a close-up now and see what this muscle is made of.

1

Myosin (thick filaments) and **actin** (thin filaments) are contained within compartments called **sarcomeres**—the functional units of skeletal muscle. During muscle contraction, myosin and actin slide over each other, reducing sarcomere length.

2

Tiny, threadlike structures called **myofibrils** run the length of the fiber and make up the fiber's bulk. Myosin and actin reside within the myofibrils.

6

The **epimysium** surrounds the entire muscle, binding all of the muscle fibers together.

3

A plasma membrane called the **sarcolemma** lies beneath the endomysium and above the nucleus.

Actin

Myosin

Nuclei

Nerve ending

Motor neuron

Bone

Tendon

4

Fibrous connective tissue called the **endomysium** surrounds each individual muscle fiber.

5

A sheath of connective tissue called the **perimysium** binds muscle fibers together into bundles called fasciculi.

Muscle attachment

Most skeletal muscles are attached to bones, either directly or indirectly.

Direct

In a direct attachment, the epimysium of the muscle fuses to the periosteum, the fibrous membrane covering the bone.

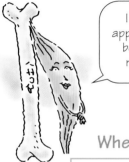

I prefer the direct approach. When I see a bone I like, I attach myself right to it.

Indirect

In an indirect attachment (most common), the epimysium extends past the muscle as a tendon, or aponeurosis, and attaches to the bone.

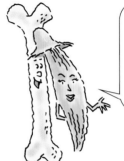

I prefer a more indirect approach. I like to slip into a tendon, and let the tendon ease me into a relationship.

Where do I begin?

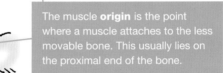

The muscle **origin** is the point where a muscle attaches to the less movable bone. This usually lies on the proximal end of the bone.

The **insertion** is the point where a muscle attaches to the more movable bone—typically on the distal end.

Muscle growth

Muscle develops when existing muscle fibers hypertrophy. Muscle strength and size differ among individuals because of such factors as:

 exercise

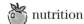 nutrition

 genetic constitution.

Changes in nutrition or exercise can alter muscle strength and size in an individual.

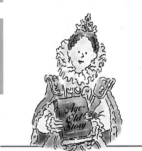

Age-old story

Aging muscles

Muscles changes associated with age include:
- decreased muscle mass
- weakness
- difficulty with tandem (heel-to-toe) walking.

Many elderly people walk with shorter steps and a wider leg stance to achieve better balance and stable weight distribution.

Muscle movements

Skeletal muscles permit several types of movement. A muscle's functional name comes from the type of movement it permits.

It's really a matter of teamwork. Most movement involves groups of muscles rather than one muscle.

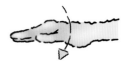

Retraction and protraction
Moving backward and forward

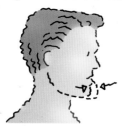

Flexion
Bending, decreasing the joint angle

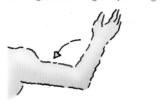

Extension
Straightening, increasing the joint angle

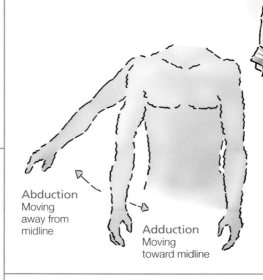

Abduction
Moving away from midline

Adduction
Moving toward midline

Pronation
Turning downward

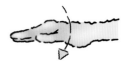

Supination
Turning upward

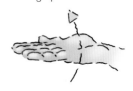

Circumduction
Moving in a circular manner

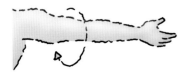

Internal rotation
Turning toward midline

External rotation
Turning away from midline

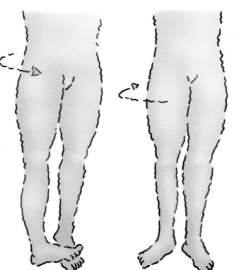

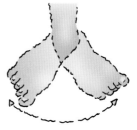

Eversion
Turning outward

Inversion
Turning inward

Muscle functions

Skeletal muscles move body parts or the body as a whole. They're responsible for both voluntary and reflex movements. Skeletal muscles also maintain posture and generate body heat. Muscles voluntarily contract when stimulated by impulses from the nervous system.

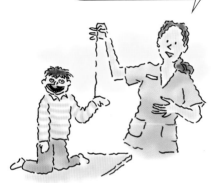

During contraction, the muscle shortens, pulling on the bone to which it's attached and applying force to the tendon.

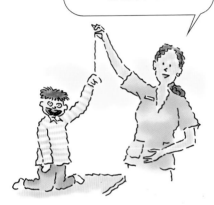

Then one bone is pulled toward, moved away from, or rotated around a second bone, depending on the type of muscle that has contracted.

Tendons and ligaments

TENDONS

attach to o

Tendons are bands of fibrous connective tissue that attach muscles to the periosteum, the fibrous covering of the bone. Tendons enable bones to move when skeletal muscles contract.

LIGAMENTS

attach to o

Ligaments are dense, strong, flexible bands of fibrous connective tissue that bind bones to other bones.

Bones

The human skeleton contains 206 bones: 80 form the axial skeleton and 126 form the appendicular skeleton.

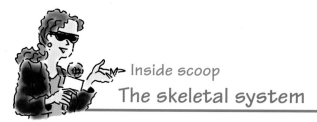

Inside scoop

The skeletal system

Bones of the axial skeleton include:
■ facial and cranial bones
■ hyoid bone
■ vertebrae
■ ribs and sternum.

Bones of the appendicular skeleton include:
■ clavicle
■ scapula
■ humerus, radius, ulna, carpals, metacarpals, and phalanges
■ pelvic bone
■ femur, patella, fibula, tibia, tarsals, metatarsals, and phalanges.

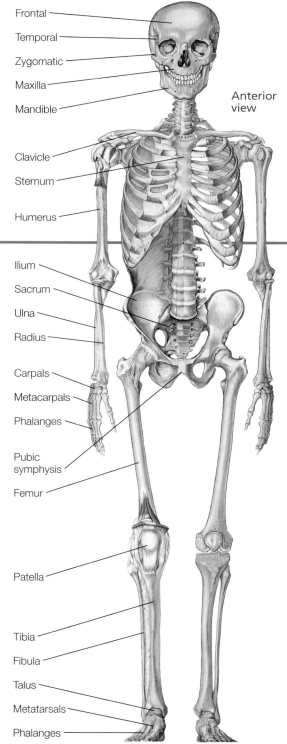

Frontal
Temporal
Zygomatic
Maxilla
Mandible

Anterior view

Clavicle
Sternum

Humerus

Ilium
Sacrum
Ulna
Radius

Carpals
Metacarpals
Phalanges

Pubic symphysis

Femur

Patella

Tibia
Fibula
Talus
Metatarsals
Phalanges

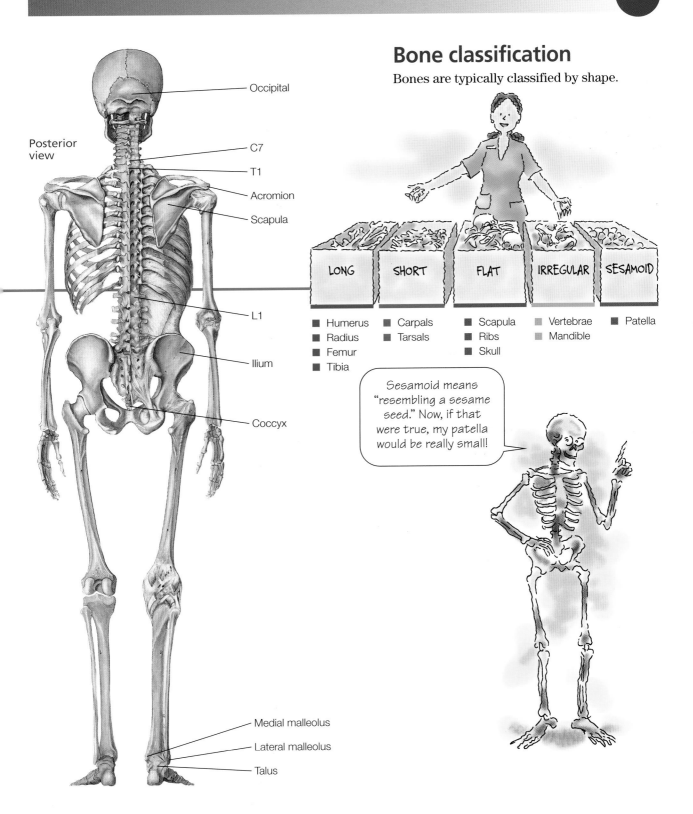

Posterior
view

Occipital

C7

T1

Acromion

Scapula

L1

Ilium

Coccyx

Medial malleolus

Lateral malleolus

Talus

Bone classification

Bones are typically classified by shape.

| LONG | SHORT | FLAT | IRREGULAR | SESAMOID |

■ Humerus   ■ Carpals   ■ Scapula   ■ Vertebrae   ■ Patella
■ Radius   ■ Tarsals   ■ Ribs   ■ Mandible
■ Femur   ■ Skull
■ Tibia

Sesamoid means
"resembling a sesame
seed." Now, if that
were true, my patella
would be really small!

Bone functions

Bones perform various anatomic (mechanical) and physiologic functions, such as:
- protect internal tissues and organs
- stabilize and support the body
- provide a surface for muscle, ligament, and tendon attachment
- move through "lever" action when contracted
- produce red blood cells in the bone marrow (a process called *hematopoiesis*)
- store mineral salts—for example, approximately 99% of the body's calcium.

Blood supply

Blood reaches bones through three paths:

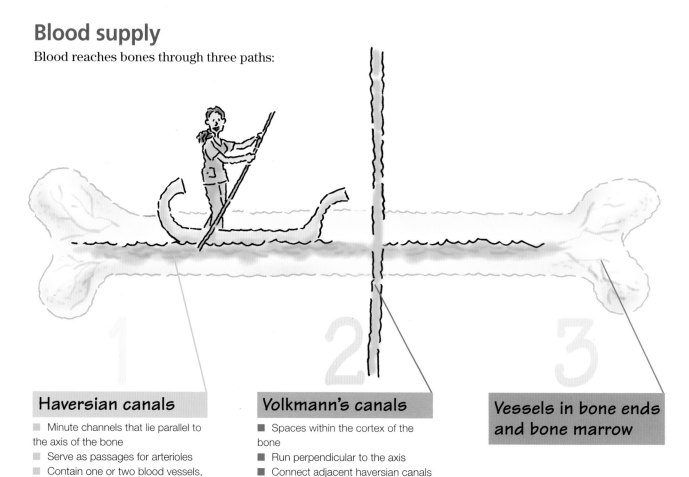

Haversian canals
- Minute channels that lie parallel to the axis of the bone
- Serve as passages for arterioles
- Contain one or two blood vessels, lymphatics, and nerve fibers

Volkmann's canals
- Spaces within the cortex of the bone
- Run perpendicular to the axis
- Connect adjacent haversian canals
- Contain blood vessels

Vessels in bone ends and bone marrow

Bone formation

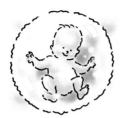

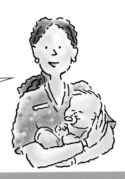

Bones begin to harden when osteoblasts (bone-forming cells) produce osteoid (a collagenous material that ossifies). This process is called *endochondral ossification*.

3 months in utero
Fetal skeleton is composed of cartilage.

6 months in utero
Fetal cartilage has been transformed into bony skeleton.

Birth
Some bones—most notably the carpals and tarsals—ossify (harden).

Bone remodeling

Two types of osteocytes—osteoblasts and osteoclasts—are responsible for remodeling.

Bone is always in a process of being created and destroyed. Now that's a big remodeling job!

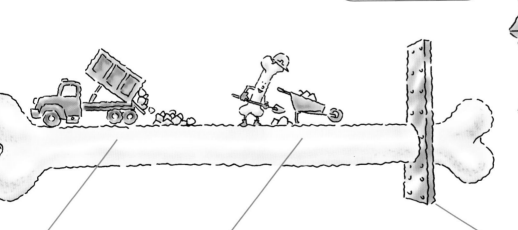

1 Osteoblasts deposit new bone.

2 Osteoclasts increase long-bone diameter. They also promote longitudinal bone growth by reabsorbing previously deposited bone.

3 Growth continues until the epiphyseal plates ossify during adolescence. (The epiphyseal plates are cartilage that separates the *diaphysis*, or shaft of a bone, from the *epiphysis*, or end of a bone.)

Cartilage

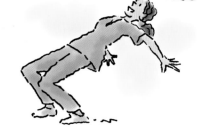

Cartilage is a dense connective tissue consisting of fibers embedded in a strong, gel-like substance. Unlike rigid bone, cartilage has the flexibility of firm plastic.

Cartilage supports and shapes various structures, such as the auditory canal and intervertebral disks. It also cushions and absorbs shock, preventing direct transmission to the bone. Cartilage has no blood supply or innervation.

Hyaline cartilage

■ Most common
■ Covers articular bone surfaces (where one or more bones meet at a joint)
■ Connects ribs to the sternum
■ Appears in the trachea, bronchi, and nasal septum

Fibrous cartilage

■ Strong and rigid
■ Composed of small quantities of matrix and abundant fibrous elements
■ Forms the symphysis pubis and intervertebral disks

Elastic cartilage

■ Elastic and resilient
■ Contains large number of elastic fibers
■ Located in the auditory canal, external ear, and epiglottis

Joints

The junction of two or more bones is called a *joint*. Joints stabilize bones and allow movement. There are two types of joints.

1 Nonsynovial

In nonsynovial joints, the bones are connected by fibrous tissue or cartilage. The bones may be immovable, like the sutures in the skull, or slightly moveable, like the vertebrae.

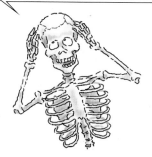

2 Synovial

In synovial joints, the bones are separate from each other and meet in a cavity filled with synovial fluid.

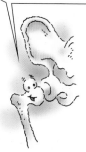

A fibrous capsule stabilizes joint structures and surrounds joint ligaments (tough, fibrous bands that join one to another).

Cartilage cushions the end of each bone.

Synovial fluid fills the joint space, allowing the joint to move freely.

Bone

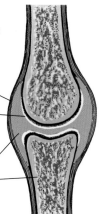

Common joints

Ball-and-socket joint

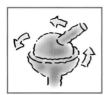

- Located in the shoulders and hips
- Allow flexion, extension, adduction, and abduction
- Rotate in their sockets
- Assessed by their degrees of internal and external rotation

Pivot joint

- Rounded portion of one bone in a pivot joint fits into a groove in another bone
- Allow only uniaxial rotation of the first bone around the second
- Includes the head of the radius, which rotates within a groove of the ulna

Hinge joint

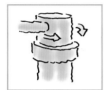

- Include the knee and the elbow
- Move in flexion and extension

Condylar joint

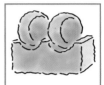

- An oval surface of one bone fits into a concavity in another bone
- Allow flexion, extension, abduction, adduction, and circumduction
- Includes the radiocarpal and metacarpophalangeal joints of the hand

Saddle joint

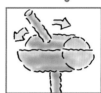

- Resemble condylar joints but allow greater freedom of movement
- Only saddle joints are the carpometacarpal joints of the thumb

Bursae

Bursae are small synovial fluid sacs located at friction points around joints between tendons, ligaments, and bones. Examples include the subacromial bursa (located in the shoulder) and the prepatellar bursa (located in the knee).

Bursae

Joint cavity

Bone

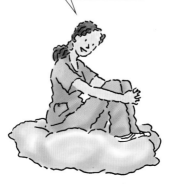

Bursae act as cushions to decrease stress on adjacent structures.

VISION QUEST

Able to label?

Label the structures of the muscle fiber shown in this illustration.

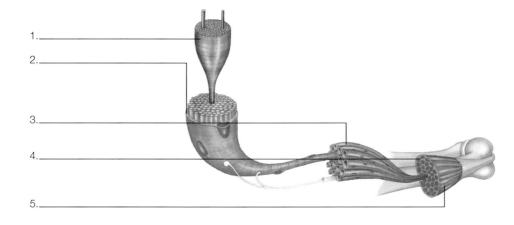

1. _____
2. _____
3. _____
4. _____
5. _____

Matchmaker

Match the five common joints types shown on the left with the movements they allow.

1. _____
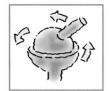

2. _____
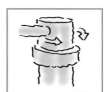

3. _____
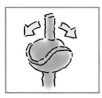

4. _____
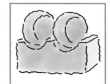

5. _____
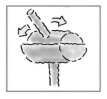

A. Allow flexion, extension, abduction, adduction, and circumduction

B. Allow flexion, extension, adduction, and abduction

C. Allow greater freedom of movement than do condylar joints

D. Move in flexion and extension

E. Allow only uniaxial rotation of the first bone around the second

6
Nervous system

● Neurons 58
● Neuroglia 59
● Central nervous system 60
● Peripheral nervous system 68
● Vision quest 70

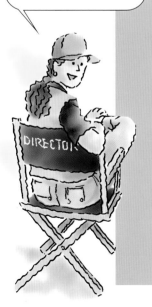

In this business, it isn't always what you know but who you know. That's why the nervous system gets a starring role: not only does it control body function, it's also related to every other body system.

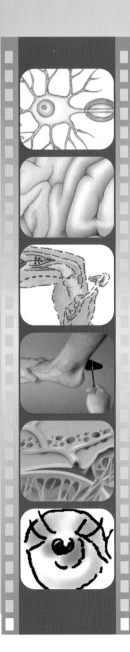

Neurons

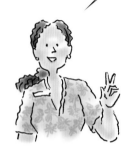

The nervous system has two main types of cells: *neurons*, which are conducting cells, and *neuroglia*, which are supportive cells.

The neuron is the basic unit of the nervous system. This highly specialized conductor cell receives and transmits electrochemical nerve impulses. Delicate, threadlike nerve fibers called *axons* and *dendrites* extend from the central cell body and transmit signals. In a typical neuron, one axon and many dendrites extend from the cell body.

You might say we neurons are the movers and shakers of this operation. After all, we receive and transmit electrochemical impulses throughout the entire nervous system. Here are some of the things that "set us off."

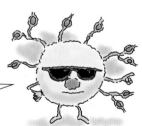

Dendrite

Cell body

Nucleus

Axon

Dendrites receive impulses from other cells and conduct them toward the cell body.

The axon conducts impulses away from the cell.

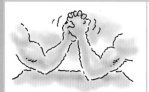

■ Mechanical stimuli (such as touch and pressure)

■ Thermal stimuli (such as heat and cold)

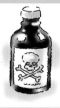

■ Chemical stimuli (either external chemicals or a chemical released by the body, such as histamine).

How neurotransmission occurs

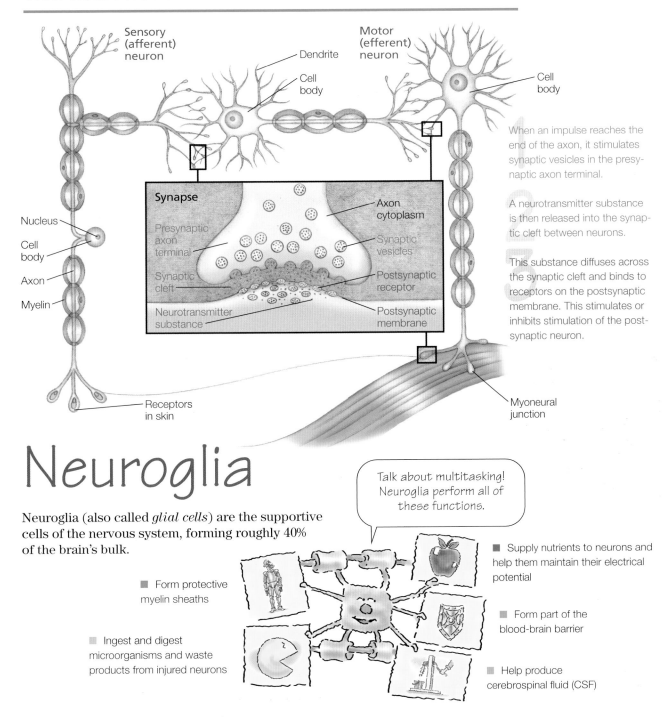

Sensory (afferent) neuron

Dendrite

Cell body

Motor (efferent) neuron

Cell body

Nucleus

Cell body

Axon

Myelin

Synapse

Presynaptic axon terminal

Synaptic cleft

Neurotransmitter substance

Axon cytoplasm

Synaptic vesicles

Postsynaptic receptor

Postsynaptic membrane

Receptors in skin

Myoneural junction

When an impulse reaches the end of the axon, it stimulates synaptic vesicles in the presynaptic axon terminal.

A neurotransmitter substance is then released into the synaptic cleft between neurons.

This substance diffuses across the synaptic cleft and binds to receptors on the postsynaptic membrane. This stimulates or inhibits stimulation of the postsynaptic neuron.

Neuroglia

Neuroglia (also called *glial cells*) are the supportive cells of the nervous system, forming roughly 40% of the brain's bulk.

Talk about multitasking! Neuroglia perform all of these functions.

■ Form protective myelin sheaths

■ Ingest and digest microorganisms and waste products from injured neurons

■ Supply nutrients to neurons and help them maintain their electrical potential

■ Form part of the blood-brain barrier

■ Help produce cerebrospinal fluid (CSF)

Central nervous system

The central nervous system includes the brain and spinal cord.

The brain

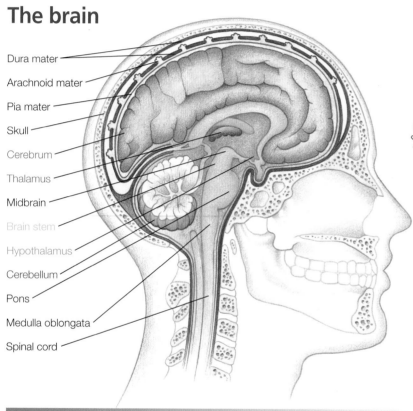

Dura mater
Arachnoid mater
Pia mater
Skull
Cerebrum
Thalamus
Midbrain
Brain stem
Hypothalamus
Cerebellum
Pons
Medulla oblongata
Spinal cord

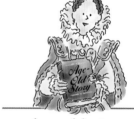

> Together with the spinal cord, I collect and interpret voluntary and involuntary motor and sensory stimuli.

Age-old story

Neurologic changes with aging

- The number of brain cells decreases at a rate of about 1% per year after age 50. (Clinical effects usually aren't noticeable until aging is more advanced.)
- The hypothalamus becomes less effective at regulating body temperature.
- The cerebral cortex undergoes a 20% neuron loss.
- Nerve transmission typically slows, resulting in a sluggish response to external stimuli.

Brain structures

Cerebrum

- Also known as *cerebral cortex*
- Controls ability to think and reason
- Enclosed by three meninges (dura mater, arachnoid mater, and pia mater)
- Contains the diencephalon, which consists of the thalamus and hypothalamus

Thalamus

- Relay station for sensory impulses

Hypothalamus

- Controls regulatory functions, including body temperature, pituitary hormone production, and water balance

Brain stem

- Regulates autonomic body functions, such as heart rate, breathing, and swallowing
- Contains cranial nerves III through XII

Cerebellum

- Contains major motor and sensory pathways
- Helps maintain equilibrium
- Controls muscle coordination

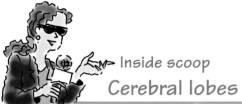

Inside scoop
Cerebral lobes

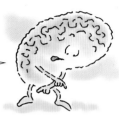

Let's see…my right hemisphere controls the left side of my body, and my left hemisphere controls the right side of my body. If I'm not careful, I'll trip over my own feet!

The cerebrum is divided into four lobes and two hemispheres.

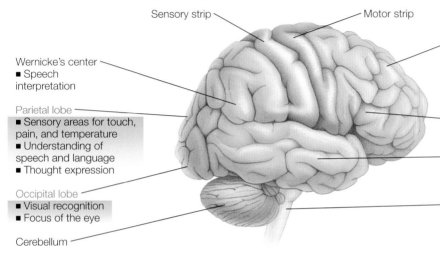

Sensory strip

Motor strip

Wernicke's center
■ Speech interpretation

Parietal lobe
■ Sensory areas for touch, pain, and temperature
■ Understanding of speech and language
■ Thought expression

Occipital lobe
■ Visual recognition
■ Focus of the eye

Cerebellum

Frontal lobe
■ Motor control of voluntary muscles
■ Personality
■ Concentration
■ Organization
■ Problem-solving

Broca's center
■ Motor control of speech

Temporal lobe
■ Hearing
■ Memory of hearing and vision

Brain stem
■ Midbrain
■ Pons
■ Medulla

Inside scoop
Limbic system

The limbic system is a primitive brain area deep within the temporal lobe. In addition to initiating basic drives (hunger, aggression, and emotional and sexual arousal), it screens all sensory messages traveling to the cerebral cortex.

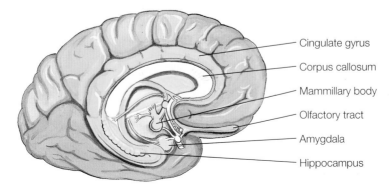

Cingulate gyrus

Corpus callosum

Mammillary body

Olfactory tract

Amygdala

Hippocampus

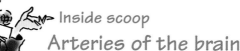

Inside scoop

Arteries of the brain

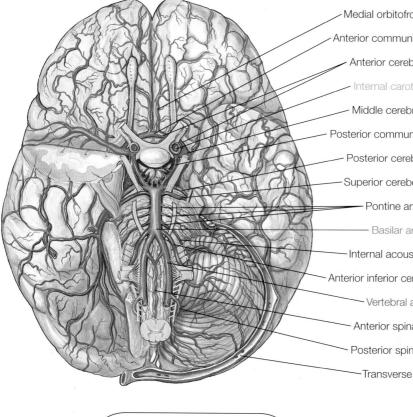

Medial orbitofrontal artery

Anterior communicating artery

Anterior cerebral artery

Internal carotid artery

Middle cerebral artery

Posterior communicating artery

Posterior cerebral artery

Superior cerebellar artery

Pontine arteries

Basilar artery

Internal acoustic artery

Anterior inferior cerebellar artery

Vertebral artery

Anterior spinal artery

Posterior spinal artery

Transverse sinus

Circle of Willis

The vertebral and carotid arteries interconnect through the circle of Willis, an anastomosis at the base of the brain. The circle of Willis ensures that oxygen is continually circulated to the brain despite interruption of any of the brain's major vessels.

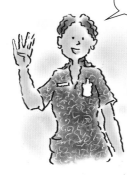

Four major arteries—two vertebral and two carotid—supply the brain with oxygenated blood.

The two vertebral arteries (branches of the subclavians) converge to become…

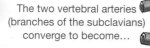

…the basilar artery, which…

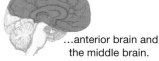

…supplies oxygen to the posterior brain.

The common carotids branch into the two internal carotids, which…

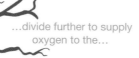

…divide further to supply oxygen to the…

…anterior brain and the middle brain.

Spinal cord

The spinal cord extends from the upper border of the first cervical vertebra to the lower border of the first lumbar vertebra. It's encased by a continuation of the meninges and CSF of the brain. It's also protected by the bony vertebrae of the spine.

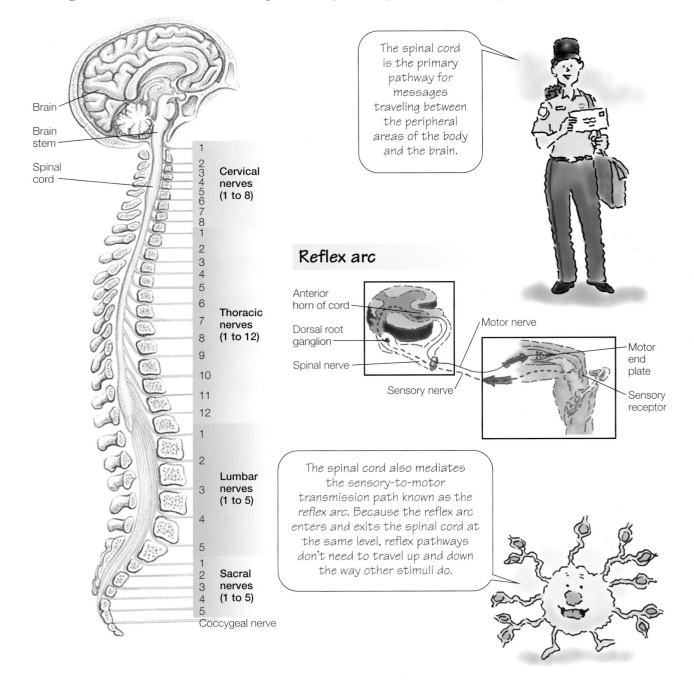

Brain

Brain stem

Spinal cord

Cervical nerves (1 to 8)

Thoracic nerves (1 to 12)

Lumbar nerves (1 to 5)

Sacral nerves (1 to 5)

Coccygeal nerve

The spinal cord is the primary pathway for messages traveling between the peripheral areas of the body and the brain.

Reflex arc

Anterior horn of cord

Dorsal root ganglion

Spinal nerve

Sensory nerve

Motor nerve

Motor end plate

Sensory receptor

The spinal cord also mediates the sensory-to-motor transmission path known as the reflex arc. Because the reflex arc enters and exits the spinal cord at the same level, reflex pathways don't need to travel up and down the way other stimuli do.

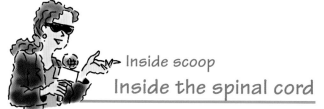

Inside scoop

Inside the spinal cord

Within the spinal cord, the H-shaped mass of gray matter is divided into horns, which consist mainly of neuron cell bodies.

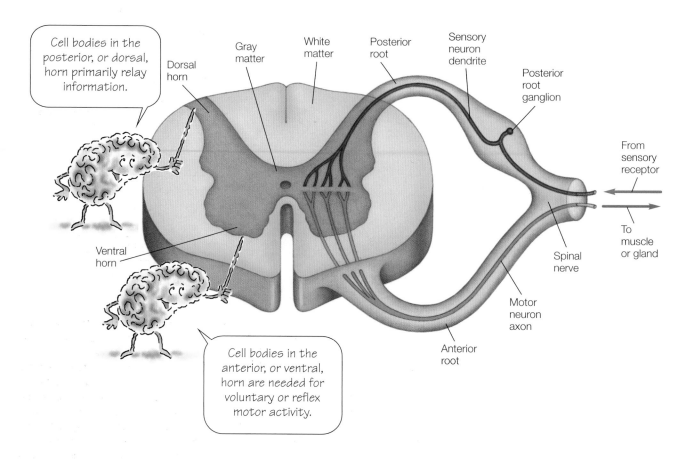

Cell bodies in the posterior, or dorsal, horn primarily relay information.

Cell bodies in the anterior, or ventral, horn are needed for voluntary or reflex motor activity.

Dorsal horn

Gray matter

White matter

Posterior root

Sensory neuron dendrite

Posterior root ganglion

From sensory receptor

To muscle or gland

Spinal nerve

Motor neuron axon

Anterior root

Ventral horn

Major neural pathways

Sensory pathways

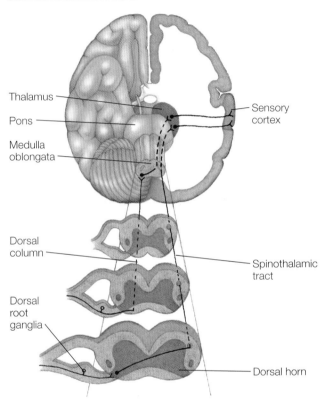

Thalamus

Pons

Medulla oblongata

Sensory cortex

Dorsal column

Spinothalamic tract

Dorsal root ganglia

Dorsal horn

Motor pathways

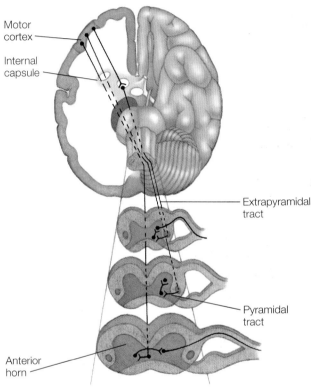

Motor cortex

Internal capsule

Extrapyramidal tract

Pyramidal tract

Anterior horn

■ Sensory impulses travel via *afferent* (sensory, or ascending) neural pathways to the sensory cortex in the parietal lobe of the brain, where they're interpreted.

■ Impulses travel up the cord in the dorsal column to the medulla, where they cross to the opposite side and enter the thalamus.

■ The thalamus then relays all incoming sensory impulses (except olfactory impulses) to the sensory cortex for interpretation.

■ Pain and temperature sensations enter the spinal cord through the dorsal horn.

■ Touch, pressure, and vibration sensations enter the cord via ganglia (knot-like masses of nerve cell bodies on the dorsal roots of spinal nerves).

Ow! The pain of that nail traveled UP my sensory pathways to my brain. My brain then sent a motor impulse DOWN to my foot telling me to jump!

■ Motor impulses travel from the brain to the muscles via the *efferent* (motor, or descending) neural pathways.

■ Motor impulses originate in the motor cortex of the frontal lobe and reach the lower motor neurons of the peripheral nervous system via upper motor neurons.

■ Upper motor neurons originate in the brain and form two major systems:
– the pyramidal system—responsible for fine, skilled movements of skeletal muscle
– the extrapyramidal system—controls gross motor movements.

Reflex responses

Reflex responses occur automatically, without any brain involvement, to protect the body. Reflex responses include:

- deep tendon reflexes—involuntary contractions of a muscle after brief stretching caused by tendon percussion
- superficial reflexes—withdrawal reflexes elicited by noxious or tactile stimulation of the skin, cornea, or mucous membranes
- primitive reflexes—abnormal in adults but normal in infants, whose central nervous systems are immature.

Eliciting deep tendon reflexes

Test deep tendon reflexes by moving from head to toe and comparing side to side.

Biceps reflex

Position the patient's arm so his elbow is flexed at a 45-degree angle and his arm is relaxed. Place your thumb or index finger over the biceps tendon. Strike your finger with the pointed end of the reflex hammer, and watch and feel for the contraction of the biceps muscle and flexion of the forearm.

Triceps reflex

Ask the patient to adduct his arm and place his forearm across his chest. Strike the triceps tendon about 2″ (5 cm) above the olecranon process on the extensor surface of the upper arm. Watch for contraction of the triceps muscle and extension of the forearm.

Patellar reflex

Ask the patient to sit with his legs dangling freely. If he can't sit up, flex his knee at a 45-degree angle and place your nondominant hand behind it for support. Strike the patellar tendon just below the patella, and look for contraction of the quadriceps muscle in the thigh with extension of the leg.

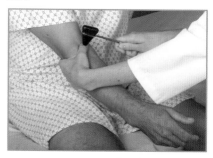

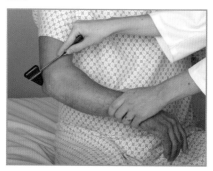

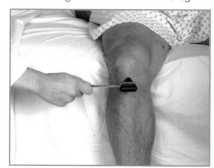

Achilles reflex

Ask the patient to flex his foot. Strike the Achilles tendon, and watch for plantar flexion of the foot at the ankle.

Brachioradialis reflex

Ask the patient to rest the ulnar surface of his hand on his abdomen or lap with the elbow partially flexed. Strike the radius, and watch for supination of the hand and flexion of the forearm at the elbow.

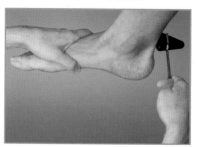

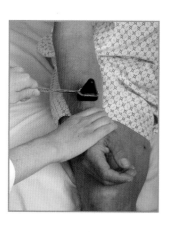

Protective structures

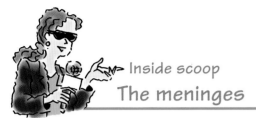

Inside scoop
The meninges

The meninges are membranous coverings that help protect the brain and spinal cord.

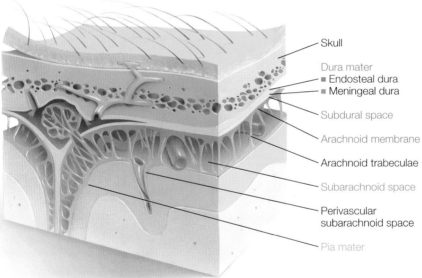

Skull

Dura mater
- Endosteal dura
- Meningeal dura

Subdural space

Arachnoid membrane

Arachnoid trabeculae

Subarachnoid space

Perivascular subarachnoid space

Pia mater

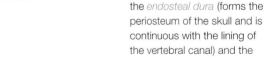

Because the spinal cord and I are important for your livelihood, we have a strong defensive team. The skull and vertebrae provide a first line of defense against shock and infection, but they can't do it alone. Here's the rest of the defensive lineup.

Defensive lineup

■ Dura mater: tough, fibrous, leatherlike tissue composed of the *endosteal dura* (forms the periosteum of the skull and is continuous with the lining of the vertebral canal) and the *meningeal dura* (a thick membrane that covers the brain, providing support and protection

■ Subdural space: lies between the dura mater and the arachnoid membrane

■ Arachnoid membrane: thin, fibrous membrane that hugs the brain and spinal cord

■ Subarachnoid space: lies between the arachnoid membrane and the pia mater

■ Pia mater: continuous, delicate layer of connective tissue that covers and contours the spinal tissue and brain

Peripheral nervous system

The peripheral nervous system consists of the peripheral nerves, cranial nerves, and autonomic nervous system.

Peripheral nerves

Peripheral sensory nerves transmit stimuli to the posterior horn of the spinal cord from sensory receptors located in the skin, muscles, sensory organs, and viscera. The area of the skin that's innervated by each sensory nerve is called a *dermatome*.

Cranial nerves

The 12 pairs of cranial nerves are the primary motor and sensory pathways between the brain, head, and neck.

Inferior view

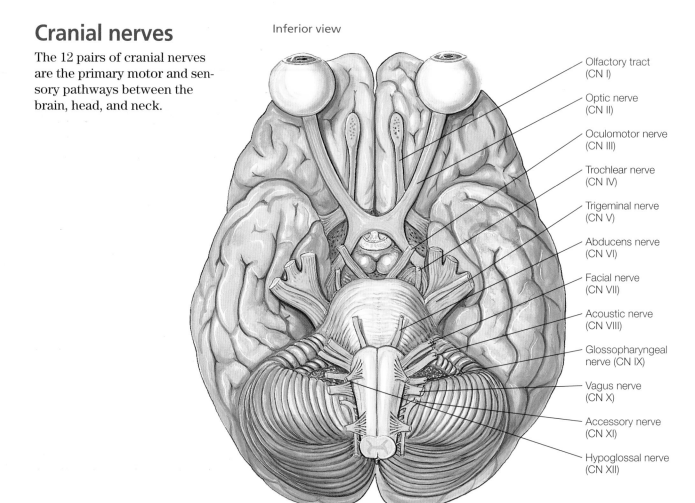

Olfactory tract (CN I)

Optic nerve (CN II)

Oculomotor nerve (CN III)

Trochlear nerve (CN IV)

Trigeminal nerve (CN V)

Abducens nerve (CN VI)

Facial nerve (CN VII)

Acoustic nerve (CN VIII)

Glossopharyngeal nerve (CN IX)

Vagus nerve (CN X)

Accessory nerve (CN XI)

Hypoglossal nerve (CN XII)

Autonomic nervous system

The autonomic nervous system controls involuntary body functions such as the activity of the cardiac muscle and glandular epithelial tissue. It has two subdivisions:

■ The sympathetic nervous system functions mainly during stress, triggering the *fight-or-flight response* (increased heart rate and respiratory rate; cold, sweaty palms; and pupil dilation).

■ The parasympathetic nervous system activates the GI system and supports restorative, resting body functions.

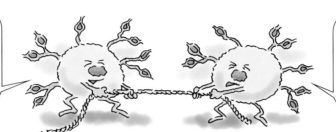

When one system stimulates a smooth muscle to contract or a gland to secrete, the other system inhibits that action.

That may seem antagonistic, but it's really designed to keep things in balance.

Effector organs	Parasympathetic responses	Sympathetic responses
Eye ■ Radial muscle of iris ■ Sphincter muscle of iris	■ None ■ Contraction for near vision	■ Contraction (mydriasis) ■ None
Heart	■ Decreased rate and contractility	■ Increased rate and contractility
Lung ■ Bronchial muscle	■ Contraction	■ Relaxation
Stomach ■ Motility and tone ■ Sphincters	■ Increased ■ Relaxation	■ Decreased (usually) ■ Contraction (usually)
Intestine ■ Motility and tone ■ Sphincters	■ Increased ■ Relaxation	■ Decreased ■ Contraction
Urinary bladder ■ Bladder muscle ■ Trigone and sphincter	■ Contraction ■ Relaxation	■ Relaxation ■ Contraction
Skin ■ Erector pili ■ Sweat glands	■ None ■ Generalized secretion	■ Contraction ■ Slight localized secretion
Adrenal medulla	■ None	■ Secretion of epinephrine and norepinephrine
Liver	■ None	■ Glycogenolysis
Pancreas ■ Acini	■ Increased secretion	■ Decreased secretion
Adipose tissue	■ None	■ Lipolysis
Juxtaglomerular cells	■ None	■ Increased renin secretion

VISION QUEST

Show and tell

Using the illustration as a guide, describe the three steps involved in neurotransmission.

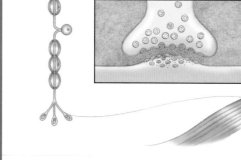

1. _____
_____
_____
_____

2. _____
_____
_____
_____

3. _____
_____
_____
_____

Matchmaker

Match each photo with the type of reflex being tested.

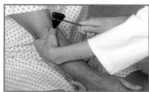 1. _____

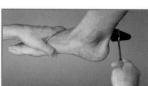 4. _____

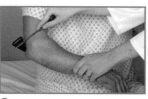 2. _____

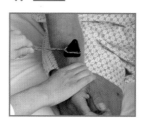 5. _____

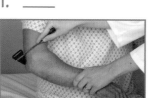 3. _____

A. Achilles
B. Biceps
C. Brachioradialis
D. Triceps
E. Patellar

70

7
Sensory system

■ The eyes 72
■ The ears 76
■ The nose 78
■ The mouth 79
■ Vision quest 80

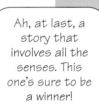

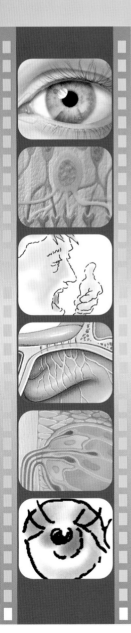

Ah, at last, a story that involves all the senses. This one's sure to be a winner!

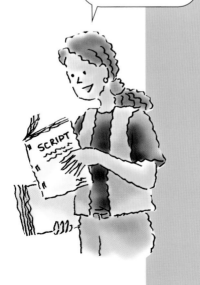

The eyes

Measuring about 1″ (2.5 cm) in diameter, eyes are sensory organs for vision. Each eye is equipped with many extraocular and intraocular structures. Some structures are easily visible, whereas others can only be viewed with special instruments.

Extraocular structures

■ Bony orbits protect the eyes from trauma.
■ The eyelids (or palpebrae) and eyelashes protect the eyes from injury, dust, and foreign bodies.
■ Conjunctivae (thin mucous membranes that line the inner surface of each eyelid and the anterior portion of the sclera) guard against invasion by foreign matter.
■ The structures of the lacrimal apparatus (lacrimal glands, punctum, lacrimal sac, and nasolacrimal duct) lubricate and protect the cornea and conjunctivae by producing and absorbing tears.
■ Extraocular muscles hold the eyes in place and control movement, helping create binocular vision.

This is no sad story. Tears also contain lysozyme, an enzyme that protects against bacterial invasion.

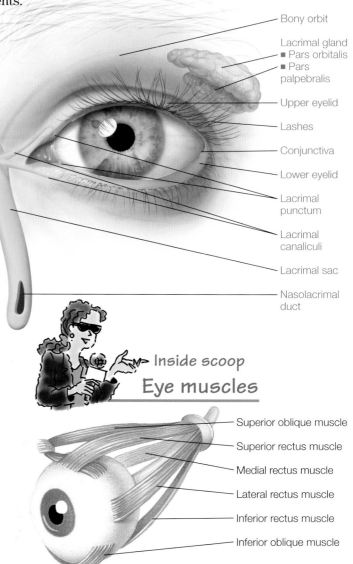

- Bony orbit
- Lacrimal gland
  - ■ Pars orbitalis
  - ■ Pars palpebralis
- Upper eyelid
- Lashes
- Conjunctiva
- Lower eyelid
- Lacrimal punctum
- Lacrimal canaliculi
- Lacrimal sac
- Nasolacrimal duct

Inside scoop
Eye muscles

- Superior oblique muscle
- Superior rectus muscle
- Medial rectus muscle
- Lateral rectus muscle
- Inferior rectus muscle
- Inferior oblique muscle

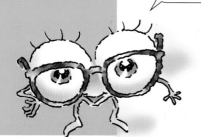

Intraocular eye structures

Anterior structures

Sclera
■ Maintains eyeball's size and shape

Conjunctiva (bulbar)

Ciliary body
■ Controls lens thickness
■ Regulates light focused onto the retina

Schlemm's canal

Iris
■ Circular contractile disk
■ Contains smooth and radial muscles

Pupil
■ Regulates light entry

Lens
■ Refracts and focuses light onto the retina

Cornea
■ Smooth, transparent tissue
■ Has no blood supply
■ Highly sensitive to touch

Anterior chamber (filled with aqueous humor)

Posterior chamber (filled with aqueous humor)

Posterior structures

Posterior sclera
■ White, opaque, fibrous layer
■ Covers the posterior segment of the eyeball

Choroid
■ Lies beneath the posterior sclera
■ Contains many small arteries and veins

Central retinal artery with vein

Optic nerve

Vitreous humor

Retina
■ Innermost layer of the eyeball
■ Receives visual stimuli and sends them to the brain

I may look good from the outside, but inside is where all the action is. My intraocular structures are directly involved with vision.

Inside scoop

A closer view of retinal structures

The retina is the innermost layer of the eyeball. It receives visual stimuli and sends them to the brain.

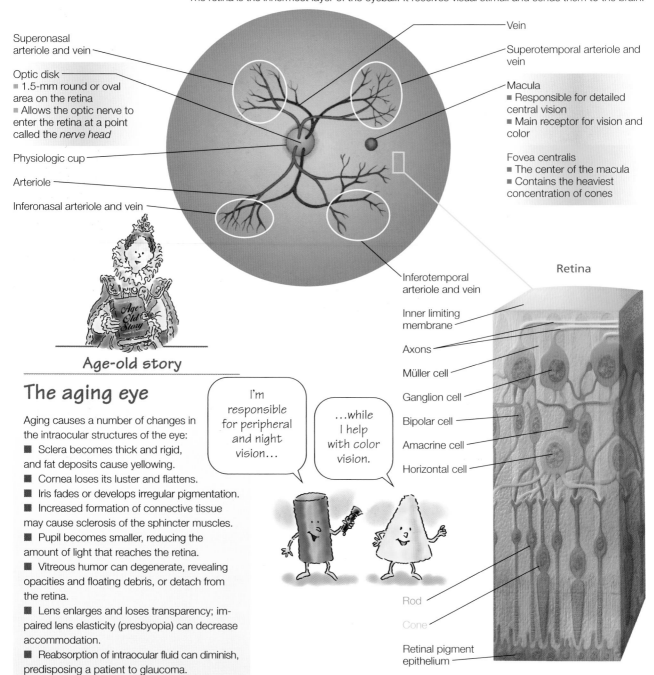

Superonasal
arteriole and vein

Optic disk
■ 1.5-mm round or oval area on the retina
■ Allows the optic nerve to enter the retina at a point called the *nerve head*

Physiologic cup

Arteriole

Inferonasal arteriole and vein

Vein

Superotemporal arteriole and vein

Macula
■ Responsible for detailed central vision
■ Main receptor for vision and color

Fovea centralis
■ The center of the macula
■ Contains the heaviest concentration of cones

Inferotemporal arteriole and vein

Retina

Inner limiting membrane

Axons

Müller cell

Ganglion cell

Bipolar cell

Amacrine cell

Horizontal cell

Rod

Cone

Retinal pigment epithelium

Age-old story

The aging eye

Aging causes a number of changes in the intraocular structures of the eye:

■ Sclera becomes thick and rigid, and fat deposits cause yellowing.
■ Cornea loses its luster and flattens.
■ Iris fades or develops irregular pigmentation.
■ Increased formation of connective tissue may cause sclerosis of the sphincter muscles.
■ Pupil becomes smaller, reducing the amount of light that reaches the retina.
■ Vitreous humor can degenerate, revealing opacities and floating debris, or detach from the retina.
■ Lens enlarges and loses transparency; impaired lens elasticity (presbyopia) can decrease accommodation.
■ Reabsorption of intraocular fluid can diminish, predisposing a patient to glaucoma.

I'm responsible for peripheral and night vision...

...while I help with color vision.

Image perception and formation

Intraocular structures receive and form images and then send them to the brain for interpretation.

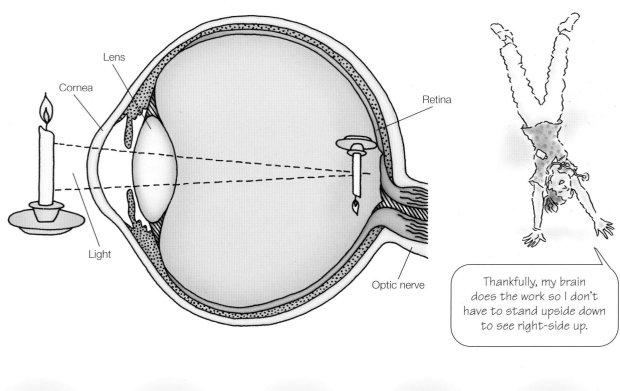

Thankfully, my brain does the work so I don't have to stand upside down to see right-side up.

1	2	3	4	5
Light shining on the cornea passes through the pupil and clear lens.	The image projected on the retina is inverted and reversed.	The rods and cones in the retina convert the light into electrical impulses.	The optic nerve collects and sends these impulses to the brain.	The brain interprets the image right side up.

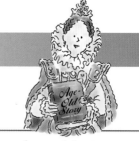

The ears

The ears are organs of hearing; they also maintain the body's equilibrium. Each ear is divided into three main parts.

Age-old story

Hearing loss

Many older people have some degree of hearing loss. One possible cause is a gradual buildup of cerumen. Another cause is a slow, progressing deafness called *presbycusis* or *senile deafness*. This irreversible, bilateral sensorineural hearing loss usually starts at middle age, slowly worsens, and affects more men than women.

External ear

The external ear collects sound.

Middle ear

The middle ear conducts sound vibrations to the inner ear.

Inner ear

The inner ear receives vibrations from the middle ear that stimulate nerve impulses. These impulses travel to the brain, and the cerebral cortex interprets the sound.

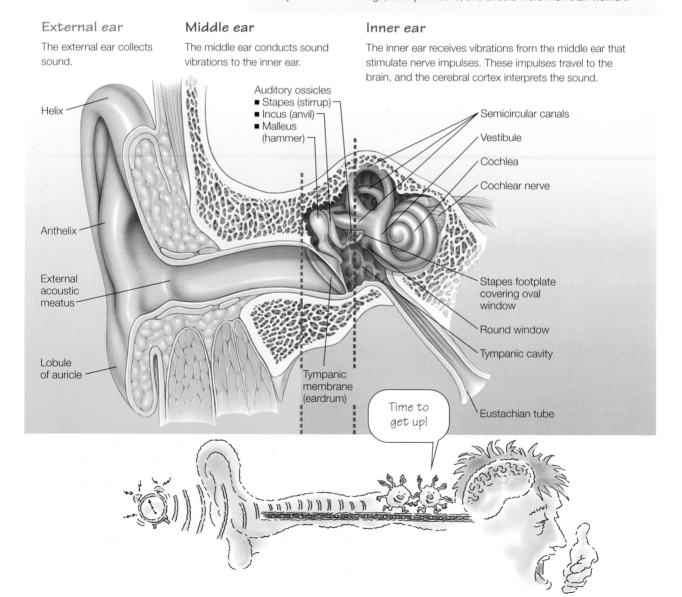

Helix

Anthelix

External acoustic meatus

Lobule of auricle

Auditory ossicles
- Stapes (stirrup)
- Incus (anvil)
- Malleus (hammer)

Tympanic membrane (eardrum)

Semicircular canals

Vestibule

Cochlea

Cochlear nerve

Stapes footplate covering oval window

Round window

Tympanic cavity

Eustachian tube

Time to get up!

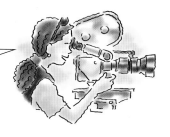

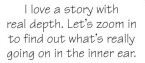

I love a story with real depth. Let's zoom in to find out what's really going on in the inner ear.

Right tympanic membrane

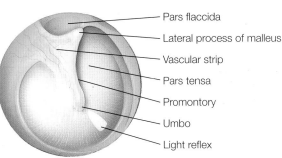

- Pars flaccida
- Lateral process of malleus
- Vascular strip
- Pars tensa
- Promontory
- Umbo
- Light reflex

Middle ear

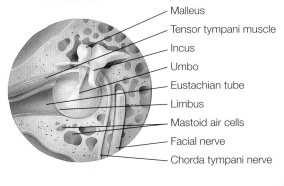

- Malleus
- Tensor tympani muscle
- Incus
- Umbo
- Eustachian tube
- Limbus
- Mastoid air cells
- Facial nerve
- Chorda tympani nerve

Membranous labyrinth
(controls sense of equilibrium and balance)

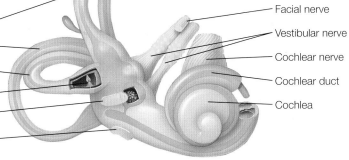

- Anterior semicircular canal
- Posterior semicircular canal
- Lateral semicircular canal
- Membranous ampulla
- Oval window
- Round window

- Facial nerve
- Vestibular nerve
- Cochlear nerve
- Cochlear duct
- Cochlea

Membranous ampulla

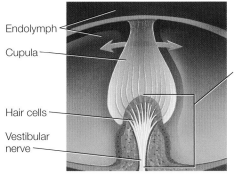

- Endolymph
- Cupula
- Crista ampullaris
- Hair cells
- Vestibular nerve

At the center of the membranous ampulla are tiny hair cells that respond to movement of fluid in the ear canals, resulting in sensations of turning or spinning.

The nose

The nose is the sense organ for smell. The mucosal epithelium that lines the uppermost portion of the nasal cavity houses receptors for fibers of the olfactory nerve (cranial nerve I). These receptors, called *olfactory (smell) receptors,* consist of hair cells that are highly sensitive but easily fatigued.

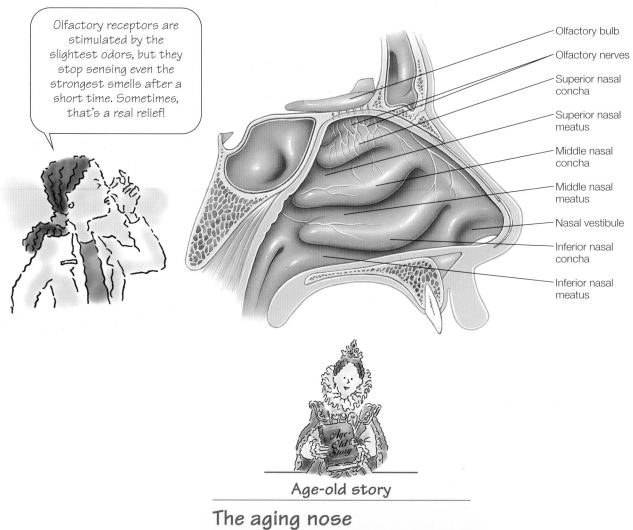

Olfactory receptors are stimulated by the slightest odors, but they stop sensing even the strongest smells after a short time. Sometimes, that's a real relief!

Olfactory bulb

Olfactory nerves

Superior nasal concha

Superior nasal meatus

Middle nasal concha

Middle nasal meatus

Nasal vestibule

Inferior nasal concha

Inferior nasal meatus

Age-old story

The aging nose

Nasal cartilage continues to grow as people age, result-ing in nose enlargement. In addition, the nasal septum—which is straight at birth and in early life—becomes slightly deviated or deformed in almost every adult.

The mouth

The roof of the mouth and the tongue contain most of the receptors for the taste nerve fibers (located in branches of cranial nerves VII and IX). Called *taste buds*, these receptors are stimulated by chemicals and respond to four taste sensations:

- sweet (on the tip of the tongue)
- sour (along the sides)
- bitter (on the back)
- salty (on the tip and sides).

All other taste sensations result when air passing through the nose stimulates olfactory receptors and taste buds.

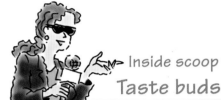

→ Inside scoop

Taste buds

Most taste buds on the tongue sit on raised protrusions of the tongue surface called *papillae*. The tongue has several types of papillae.

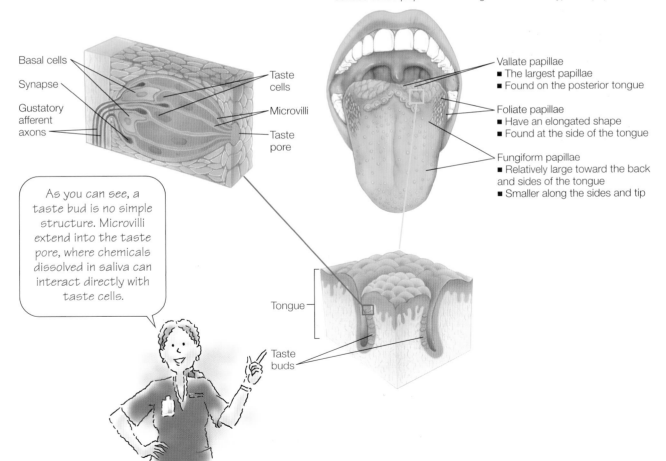

Basal cells

Synapse

Gustatory afferent axons

Taste cells

Microvilli

Taste pore

Vallate papillae
- The largest papillae
- Found on the posterior tongue

Foliate papillae
- Have an elongated shape
- Found at the side of the tongue

Fungiform papillae
- Relatively large toward the back and sides of the tongue
- Smaller along the sides and tip

As you can see, a taste bud is no simple structure. Microvilli extend into the taste pore, where chemicals dissolved in saliva can interact directly with taste cells.

Tongue

Taste buds

VISION QUEST

Able to label?

Identify the intraocular structures shown on this illustration.

1. _____
2. _____
3. _____
4. _____
5. _____
6. _____
7. _____

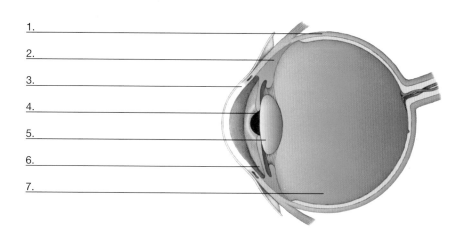

Show and tell

Using the illustration as a guide, describe the process of image perception and formation.

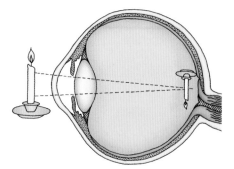

1. _____

2. _____

3. _____

4. _____

5. _____

Answers: Able to label? 1. Sclera, 2. Ciliary body, 3. Cornea, 4. Pupil, 5. Lens, 6. Iris, 7. Vitreous humor. Show and tell: 1. Light shining on the cornea passes through the pupil and clear lens. 2. The image projected on the retina is inverted and reversed. 3. The rods and cones in the retina convert the light into electrical impulses. 4. The optic nerve collects and sends these impulses to the brain. 5. The brain interprets the image right side up.

8
Endocrine system

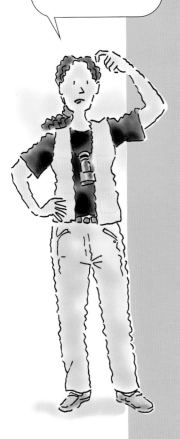

Instead of influencing people to make projects happen, the endocrine system influences organs to make body processes happen! Is life imitating art or art imitating life?

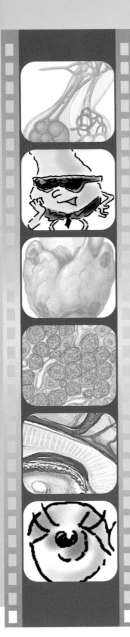

- Glands 82
- Hormones 88
- Receptors 91
- Vision quest 92

Glands

Endocrine glands secrete hormones directly into the bloodstream to regulate body function. This illustration shows the location of the major endocrine glands.

The three major components of the endocrine system are glands, hormones, and receptors.

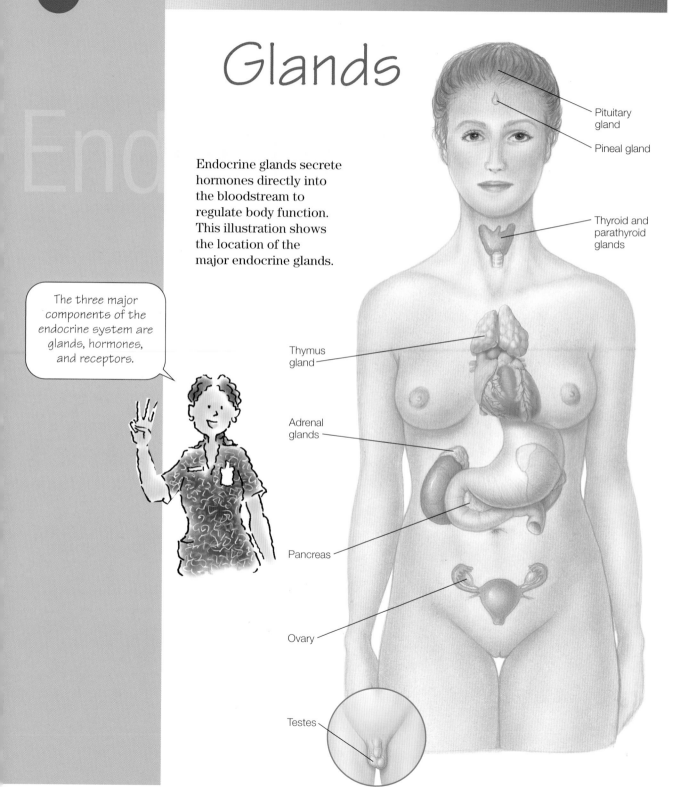

Pituitary gland

Pineal gland

Thyroid and parathyroid glands

Thymus gland

Adrenal glands

Pancreas

Ovary

Testes

Pituitary gland

The pituitary, a pea-sized gland, rests in the sella turcica, a depression in the sphenoid bone at the base of the brain.

> I may be small, but I'm a gland of great influence. I produce a number of hormones and factors to inhibit or stimulate other endocrine glands.

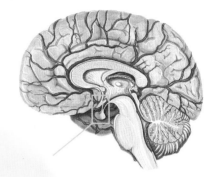

Hypothalamus

Neural pathway connecting hypothalamus to the posterior pituitary

Anterior pituitary

- Also called the *adenohypophysis*
- Is the larger of the two regions
- Produces numerous hormones, including:
  – Growth hormone (GH)
  – Prolactin
  – Thyroid-stimulating hormone (TSH)
  – Adrenocorticotropic hormone (ACTH)
  – Follicle-stimulating hormone (FSH)
  – Luteinizing hormone (LH)
  – Melanocyte-stimulating hormone (MSH)

Posterior pituitary

- Makes up about 25% of the gland
- Serves as a storage area for antidiuretic hormone (ADH), or vasopressin, and oxytocin, which are produced by the hypothalamus
- Secretes ADH and oxytocin in response to hypothalamic stimulation

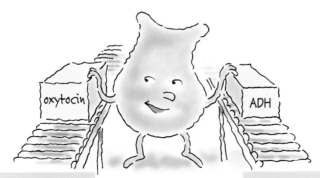

Oxytocin stimulates uterine contractions during labor and milk secretion in lactating women.

ADH stimulates the body to retain water.

Thyroid and parathyroid glands

The thyroid, a butterfly-shaped gland, lies directly below the larynx, partially in front of the trachea.

Now, these are my kinds of glands! Both help regulate blood calcium levels: the thyroid gland secretes calcitonin to inhibit the release of calcium from bone, while parathyroid hormone adjusts the rate of calcium and magnesium ion loss in urine.

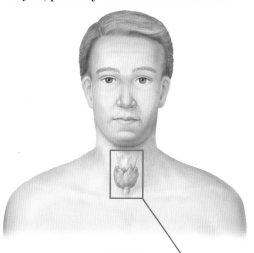

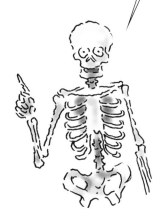

Thyroid gland

- Has two lobes that function as one unit
- Produces the hormones *thyroxine* (T_4) and *triiodothyronine* (T_3)
  - Collectively referred to as thyroid hormone
  - Body's major metabolic hormone
  - Regulates metabolism by speeding cellular respiration
- Also produces *calcitonin*
  - Maintains blood calcium level by inhibiting the release of calcium from bone
  - Alters secretion according to the calcium concentration in surrounding fluid

Superior parathyroids

Thyroid cartilage

Parathyroid glands

- Smallest known endocrine glands
- Embedded on the posterior surface of the thyroid (one in each corner)
- Work together as a single gland
- Produce *parathyroid hormone* (PTH)
  - Helps regulate blood's calcium balance by adjusting the rate at which calcium and magnesium ions are removed from urine
  - Increases movement of phosphate ions from the blood to urine for excretion

Isthmus

Trachea

Inferior parathyroids

Adrenal glands

The two adrenal glands each lie on top of a kidney. These almond-shaped glands contain two distinct structures—the adrenal cortex and the adrenal medulla—that function as separate endocrine glands.

Because catecholamines play an important role in the autonomic nervous system, the adrenal medulla is considered a neuroendocrine structure.

Adrenal cortex

- Forms the bulk of the adrenal gland
- Consists of three zones, or cell layers
  - Zona glomerulosa
  - Zona fasciculata
  - Zona reticularis
- Zones produce:
  - mineralocorticoids (primarily aldosterone)
  - glucocorticoids (cortisol [hydrocortisone], cortisone, and corticosterone)
  - small amounts of the sex hormones androgen and estrogen

Capsule

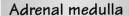

Adrenal medulla

- Functions as part of the sympathetic nervous system
- Produces two catecholamines

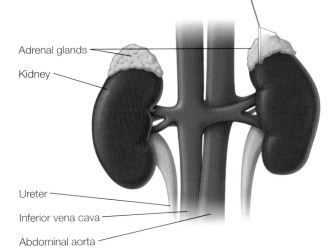

Adrenal glands

Kidney

Ureter

Inferior vena cava

Abdominal aorta

Pancreas

Nestled in the curve of the duodenum, the pancreas stretches horizontally behind the stomach and extends to the spleen. It performs both *endocrine* (inward secretion) and *exocrine* (outward secretion) functions.

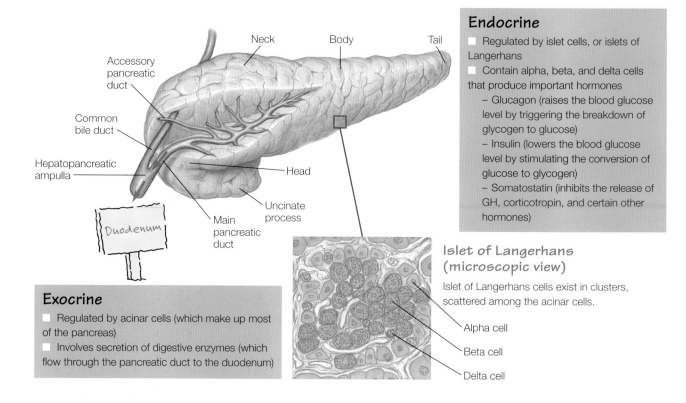

Endocrine

- ☐ Regulated by islet cells, or islets of Langerhans
- ☐ Contain alpha, beta, and delta cells that produce important hormones
  - Glucagon (raises the blood glucose level by triggering the breakdown of glycogen to glucose)
  - Insulin (lowers the blood glucose level by stimulating the conversion of glucose to glycogen)
  - Somatostatin (inhibits the release of GH, corticotropin, and certain other hormones)

Islet of Langerhans (microscopic view)

Islet of Langerhans cells exist in clusters, scattered among the acinar cells.

Alpha cell
Beta cell
Delta cell

Exocrine

- ☐ Regulated by acinar cells (which make up most of the pancreas)
- ☐ Involves secretion of digestive enzymes (which flow through the pancreatic duct to the duodenum)

Pancreatic secretions

Secretions from the pancreas assist with the digestion of many substances. This chart summarizes the functions of enzymes contained in the pancreatic secretions.

Enzyme	Function
Trypsin, chymotrypsin, and carboxypeptidase	Digest protein
Ribonuclease and deoxyribonuclease	Digest nucleic acids
Amylase	Digests starch
Lipase	Digests fats and other lipids
Cholesterol esterase	Splits cholesterol esters into cholesterol and fatty acids

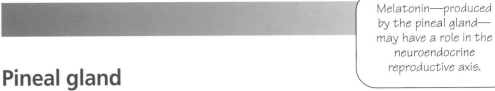

Melatonin—produced by the pineal gland—may have a role in the neuroendocrine reproductive axis.

Pineal gland

The tiny pinecone-shaped gland lies at the back of the third ventricle of the brain. It produces the hormone melatonin, which has many widespread effects.

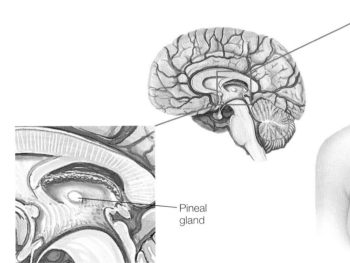

Pineal gland

Thymus

Located below the sternum and between the lungs, the thymus contains primarily lymphatic tissue. It reaches maximum size at puberty and then starts to atrophy.

Right lobe

Left lobe

Because it produces T cells, the thymus gland's major role seems to be related to the immune system.

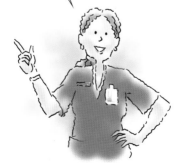

Thymus gland

- Produces T cells (important in cell-mediated immunity)
- Produces the peptide hormones thymosin and thymopoietin (promote growth of peripheral lymphoid tissue)

Gonads

Ovaries

☐ Paired, oval glands situated on either side of the uterus

☐ Produce ova (eggs) and the steroidal hormones estrogen and progesterone

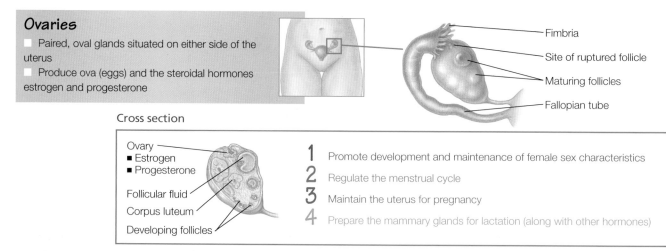

- Fimbria
- Site of ruptured follicle
- Maturing follicles
- Fallopian tube

Cross section

Ovary
- Estrogen
- Progesterone

Follicular fluid

Corpus luteum

Developing follicles

1 Promote development and maintenance of female sex characteristics

2 Regulate the menstrual cycle

3 Maintain the uterus for pregnancy

4 Prepare the mammary glands for lactation (along with other hormones)

Testes

☐ Paired structures that lie in the scrotum

☐ Produce spermatozoa and the male sex hormone testosterone (stimulates and maintains male sex characteristics)

Cross section

Epididymis

Efferent ducts of epididymis

Seminiferous tubule

Leydig cells

Microscopic view

Hormones

Hormones are complex chemicals that trigger or regulate the activity of an organ or a group of cells.

Classification of hormones

Hormones are classified by their molecular structure as polypeptides, steroids, or amines.

Classification	Hormones
Polypeptides Made of many amino acids connected by peptide bonds	■ Anterior pituitary hormones (GH, TSH, FSH, LH, and prolactin) ■ Posterior pituitary hormones (ADH and oxytocin) ■ Parathyroid hormone (PTH) ■ Pancreatic hormones (insulin and glucagon)
Steroids Derived from cholesterol	■ Adrenocortical hormones (aldosterone and cortisol) ■ Sex hormones (estrogen and progesterone in females and testosterone in males)
Amines Derived from tyrosine	■ Thyroid hormones (T_4 and T_3) ■ Catecholamines (epinephrine, norepinephrine, and dopamine)

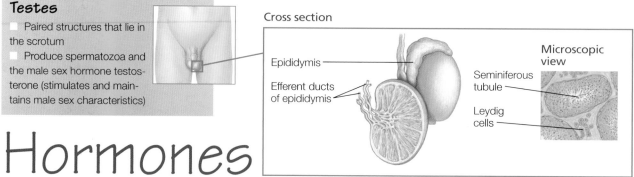

> When a hormone reaches its target site, it binds to a specific receptor on the cell membrane or within the cell.

Hormone release and transport

Although all hormone release results from endocrine gland stimulation, release patterns of hormones vary greatly.

Hormone action

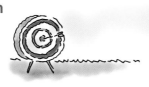

Right on target

■ Polypeptides and some amines bind to membrane receptor sites.
■ Smaller, more lipid-soluble steroids and thyroid hormones diffuse through the cell membrane and bind to intracellular receptors.
■ After binding occurs, each hormone produces unique physiologic changes, depending on its target site and its specific action at that site.
■ A particular hormone may exert different effects at different target sites.

Hormone regulation

To maintain the body's delicate equilibrium, a feedback mechanism regulates hormone production and secretion. The mechanism involves hormones, blood chemicals and metabolites, and the nervous system. This system may be simple or complex.

> One substance regulates the secretion of one hormone...simple!

> Two glands and two substances affect the secretion of one hormone...complex!

Simple feedback

Serum Ca$^+$ level ▼

Serum Ca$^+$ level ▲

Inhibits secretion of PTH

Stimulates parathyroid gland to secrete PTH

Promotes absorption of Ca+ from the GI tract, kidneys, and bone

Complex feedback

Complex feedback occurs through an axis established between the hypothalamus, pituitary gland, and target organ.

Hypothalamus secretes corticotropin-releasing hormone

Secretion of corticotropin-releasing hormone ▼

Serum cortisol level ▲

Corticotropin secretion ▼

Stimulates pituitary to secrete corticotropin

Stimulates adrenal gland to secrete cortisol

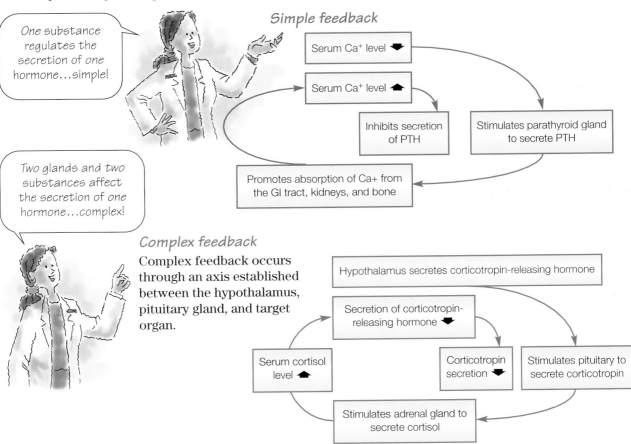
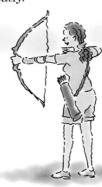

Mechanisms that control hormone release

Four basic mechanisms control hormone release.

1 Pituitary-target gland axis

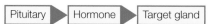

The pituitary gland regulates other endocrine glands by releasing and inhibiting hormones. These hormones include:
- corticotropin, which regulates adrenocortical hormones
- TSH, which regulates T_4 and T_3
- LH, which regulates gonadal hormones.

The pituitary continuously monitors levels of hormones produced by its target glands. If a change occurs, the pituitary corrects it by increasing or decreasing the trophic hormones.

2 Hypothalamic-pituitary-target gland axis

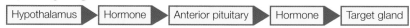

The hypothalamus also produces trophic hormones that regulate anterior pituitary hormones. By controlling anterior pituitary hormones, which regulate the target gland hormones, the hypothalamus affects target glands as well.

3 Chemical regulation

Blood glucose level ▷ Target gland

Endocrine glands not controlled by the pituitary gland may be controlled by specific substances that trigger gland secretions. For example, blood glucose level is a major regulator of glucagon and insulin release.

4 Nervous system regulation

The central nervous system (CNS) helps to regulate hormone secretion in several ways.

- Hypothalamic nerve cells stimulate the posterior pituitary to produce ADH and oxytocin. Therefore, these hormones are controlled directly by the CNS.

Hypothalamic nerve cells ▷ Posterior pituitary ▷ ADH and oxytocin

- Nervous system stimuli—such as hypoxia (oxygen deficiency), nausea, pain, stress, and certain drugs—also affect ADH levels.

Nervous system stimuli ▷ ADH

- The autonomic nervous system (ANS) controls catecholamine secretion by the adrenal medulla.

ANS ▷ Adrenal medulla ▷ Catecholamines

- The nervous system also affects other endocrine hormones. For example, stress, which leads to sympathetic stimulation, causes the pituitary to release corticotropin.

Stress ▷ Sympathetic nervous system ▷ Pituitary ▷ Corticotropin

Receptors

Receptors are protein molecules that bind specifically with other molecules, such as hormones, to trigger specific physiologic changes in a target cell.

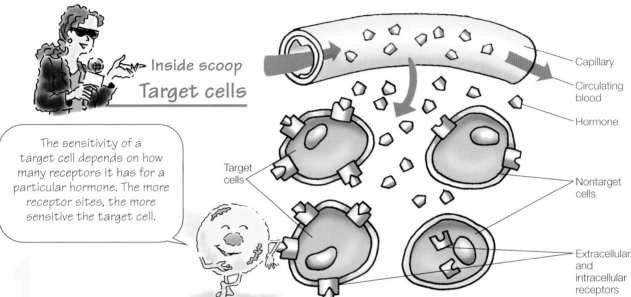

Inside scoop
Target cells

Capillary

Circulating blood

Hormone

Target cells

Nontarget cells

Extracellular and intracellular receptors

> The sensitivity of a target cell depends on how many receptors it has for a particular hormone. The more receptor sites, the more sensitive the target cell.

1

When released, a hormone travels to target cells.

2

Cells that have receptors specific to that hormone recognize the hormone and bind to it. A hormone acts only on cells with receptors specific to that hormone.

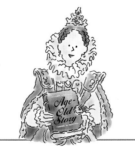

Age-old story

> For normal function, each gland must contain enough appropriately programmed secretory cells to release active hormone on demand.

> We can't do it alone, though. We receive signals telling us when to release a hormone and how much to release.

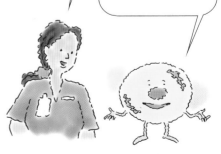

Age-related endocrine changes

As a person ages, normal changes in endocrine function include:
- reduced progesterone production
- a 50% decline in serum aldosterone levels
- a 25% decrease in cortisol secretion rate.

Also, under stressful conditions, an elderly person's blood glucose level rises higher and remains elevated longer than does a younger adult's.

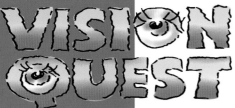

Able to label?

Identify the structures of the endocrine system shown on these illustrations.

1. _____
2. _____
3. _____
4. _____
5. _____
6. _____
7. _____
8. _____

My word!

Use the clues to help you unscramble the names of some of the body's major glands. Then use the circled letters to answer the question posed.

Question: What chemical substance triggers or regulates the activity of an organ or group of cells?

1. Serves as storage area for ADH

   poetorris tauipitry

   — ◯ — — ◯ — — — —   — — — — — — — — ◯ —

2. Part of almond-shaped gland that sits on top of the kidney

   leadran dualelm

   — — — — ◯ — —   ◯ — — — — — —

3. Has two lobes that function as one unit

   dryhoit   — ◯ — — ◯ — —

Answer: _ _ _ _ _ _ _ _

9 Cardiovascular system

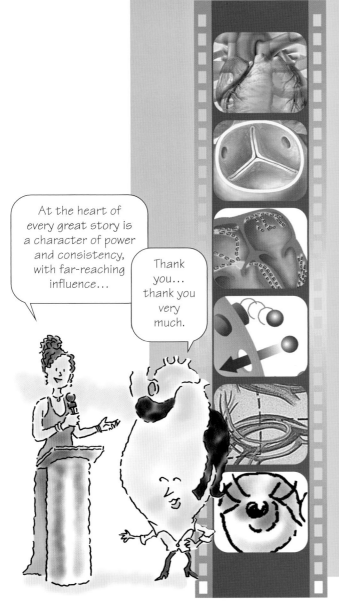

At the heart of every great story is a character of power and consistency, with far-reaching influence...

Thank you... thank you very much.

- Location of the heart 94
- Structures of the heart 95
- Flow of blood through the heart 98
- Cardiac conduction 99
- Cardiac output 101
- Arteriovenous circulation 102
- Specialized circulatory systems 104
- Vision quest 106

Location of the heart

The heart lies beneath the sternum within the mediastinum, a cavity that also contains the great vessels and trachea. In most people, two-thirds of the heart extends to the left of the body's midline, close to the left midclavicular line. The heart rests obliquely so that its broad part (the base) is at its upper right and the pointed end (the apex) is at its lower left. The apex is the point of maximal impulse, where heart sounds are loudest.

Sure I lean to the left, but I'm really politically neutral.

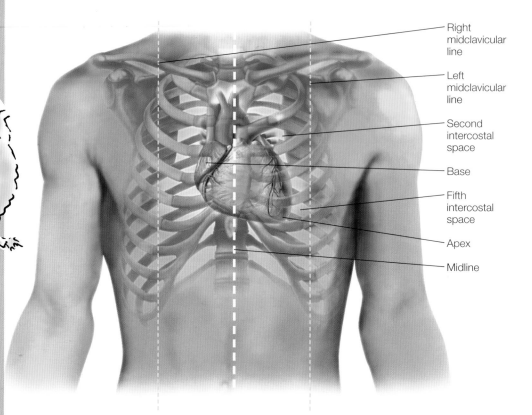

Right midclavicular line

Left midclavicular line

Second intercostal space

Base

Fifth intercostal space

Apex

Midline

Structures of the heart

Heart wall layers

■ The epicardium, the outer layer, is made up of squamous epithelial cells verlying connective tissue.
■ The myocardium, the middle layer, forms most of the heart wall. It has striated muscle fibers that cause the heart to contract.
■ The endocardium, the heart's inner layer, consists of endothelial tissue with small blood vessels and bundles of smooth muscle.

Pericardium

A sac called the *pericardium* surrounds the heart and roots of the great vessels. It consists of two layers: the fibrous pericardium (tough, white fibrous tissue) and serous pericardium (thin, smooth inner portion). The serous pericardium also has two layers: the parietal layer (lines the inside of the fibrous pericardium) and the visceral layer (adheres to the surface of the heart).

Between the fibrous and serous pericardium is the pericardial space. This space contains pericardial fluid (10 to 20 ml), which lubricates the surfaces of the space and allows the heart to move easily during contraction.

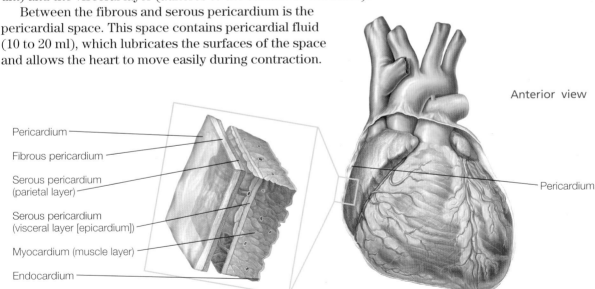

Anterior view

Pericardium

Fibrous pericardium

Serous pericardium (parietal layer)

Serous pericardium (visceral layer [epicardium])

Myocardium (muscle layer)

Endocardium

Pericardium

Heart chambers

Within the heart lie four hollow chambers: two atria and two ventricles.

■ The right and left atria serve as volume reservoirs for blood being sent into the ventricles.

– The interatrial septum divides the atrial chambers, helping them to contract and force blood into the ventricles below.

■ The ventricles serve as the pumping chambers of the heart.

– The interventricular septum separates the ventricles and also helps them to pump.

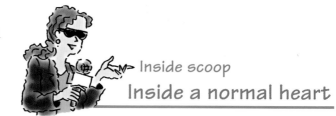

Inside scoop

Inside a normal heart

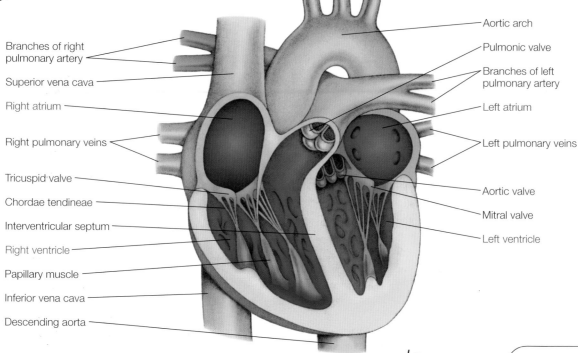

Branches of right pulmonary artery

Superior vena cava

Right atrium

Right pulmonary veins

Tricuspid valve

Chordae tendineae

Interventricular septum

Right ventricle

Papillary muscle

Inferior vena cava

Descending aorta

Aortic arch

Pulmonic valve

Branches of left pulmonary artery

Left atrium

Left pulmonary veins

Aortic valve

Mitral valve

Left ventricle

Pump it up!

The thickness of a chamber's wall depends on the amount of high-pressure work the chamber does:

■ Because the atria only have to pump blood into the ventricles, their walls are relatively thin.

■ The walls of the **right ventricle** are thicker because it pumps blood against the resistance of the pulmonary circulation.

■ The walls of the **left ventricle** are thickest of all because it pumps blood against the resistance of the systemic circulation.

The more a muscle works, the larger it becomes.

Heart valves

The heart contains four valves: two atrioventricular (AV) valves (the mitral and tricuspid) and two semilunar valves (the pulmonic and aortic). The valves allow forward flow of blood through the heart and prevent backward flow.

The tricuspid valve, or right AV valve, prevents backflow from the right ventricle into the right atrium. The mitral valve, also known as the *bicuspid* or *left AV valve*, prevents backflow from the left ventricle into the left atrium. The pulmonic valve, one of the two semilunar valves, prevents backflow from the pulmonary artery into the right ventricle. The other semilunar valve is the aortic valve, which prevents backflow from the aorta into the left ventricle.

Top view

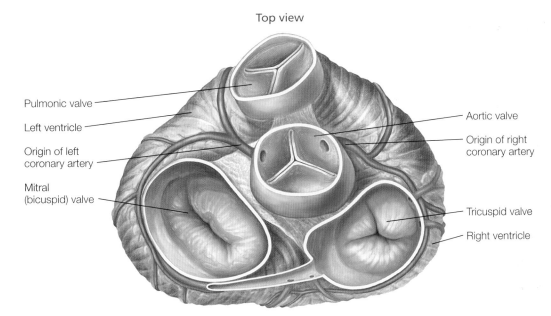

Pulmonic valve

Left ventricle

Origin of left coronary artery

Mitral (bicuspid) valve

Aortic valve

Origin of right coronary artery

Tricuspid valve

Right ventricle

The valves open to allow forward flow of blood through the heart. They immediately snap closed to prevent backward flow.

SNAP

Under pressure!

Pressure changes within the heart affect the opening and closing of the valves. The amount of blood stretching the chamber and the degree of contraction of the chamber wall determine the pressure. For example, as blood fills a chamber, the pressure rises; then, as the chamber wall contracts, the pressure rises further. This increase in pressure causes the valve to open and blood to flow out into an area of lower pressure, leading to an equal pressure state.

Flow of blood through the heart

Just like dancing a waltz, blood follows specific steps as it flows through the heart. One, two, three; one, two, three...

Step 1

Blood fills all heart chambers. The right atrium receives deoxygenated blood returning from the body through the inferior and superior vena cavae and from the heart through the coronary sinus. The left atrium receives oxygenated blood from the lungs through the four pulmonary veins. Passive filling of the ventricles begins with diastole.

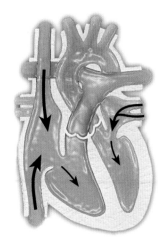

Step 2

The atria contract. The remaining blood enters the ventricles. The atria pump their blood through the two AV valves (mitral and tricuspid) directly into their respective ventricles.

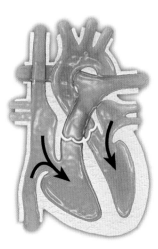

Step 3

The ventricles contract. Blood enters the aorta and pulmonary arteries. The right ventricle pumps blood through the pulmonic valve into the pulmonary arteries and then into the lungs. That blood returns, oxygenated, to the left atrium, completing pulmonic circulation.

The left ventricle pumps blood through the aortic valve into the aorta and then throughout the body. Deoxygenated blood returns to the right atrium, completing systemic circulation.

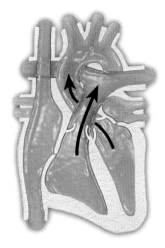

Cardiac conduction

The conduction system of the heart begins with the heart's pacemaker: the sinoatrial (SA) node. When an impulse leaves the **SA node,** it travels through the atria along **Bachmann's bundle** and the **internodal pathways** on its way to the AV node. After the impulse passes through the **AV node,** it travels to the ventricles, first down the **bundle of His,** then along the **bundle branches** and, finally, down the **Purkinje fibers.**

> The firing of the SA node sets off a chain reaction in cardiac conduction.

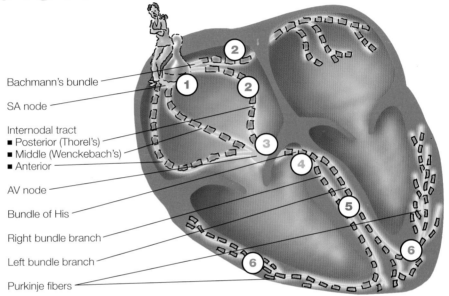

Bachmann's bundle

SA node

Internodal tract
- Posterior (Thorel's)
- Middle (Wenckebach's)
- Anterior

AV node

Bundle of His

Right bundle branch

Left bundle branch

Purkinje fibers

Pacemakers of the heart

The SA node is the heart's primary pacemaker. Pacemaker cells in lower areas, such as the junctional tissue and the Purkinje fibers, initiate an impulse only when they don't receive one from above, such as when the SA node is damaged from a myocardial infarction.

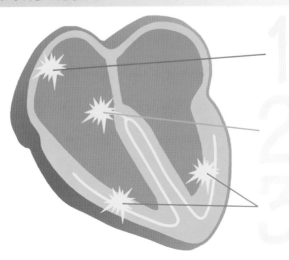

SA node
The SA node has a firing rate of 60 to 100 beats/minute.

AV node
The AV node has a firing rate of 40 to 60 beats/minute.

Purkinje fibers
The Purkinje fibers have a firing rate of 20 to 40 beats/minute.

Generation and transmission of electrical impulses depend on four characteristics of cardiac cells.

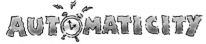 **AUTOMATICITY** ability to spontaneously initiate an impulse (pacemaker cells have this ability)

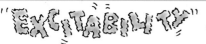 **EXCITABILITY** a cell's response to an electrical stimulus (results from ion shifts across the cell membrane)

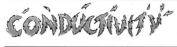 **CONDUCTIVITY** ability of a cell to transmit an electrical impulse to another cardiac cell

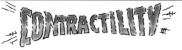 **CONTRACTILITY** ability of a cell to contract after receiving a stimulus

Depolarization-repolarization cycle

As impulses are transmitted, cardiac cells undergo cycles of depolarization and repolarization. The depolarization-repolarization cycle has five phases.

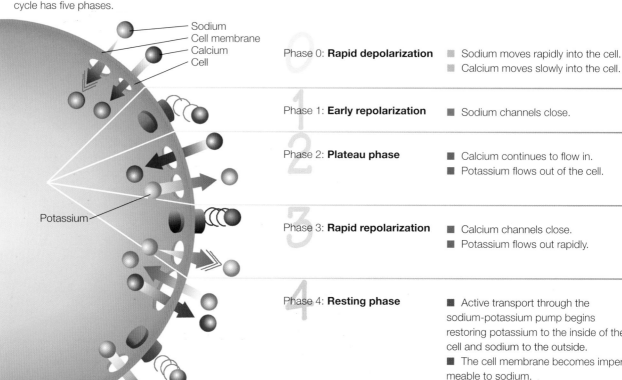

Sodium
Cell membrane
Calcium
Cell

Potassium

Phase 0: **Rapid depolarization**
■ Sodium moves rapidly into the cell.
■ Calcium moves slowly into the cell.

Phase 1: **Early repolarization**
■ Sodium channels close.

Phase 2: **Plateau phase**
■ Calcium continues to flow in.
■ Potassium flows out of the cell.

Phase 3: **Rapid repolarization**
■ Calcium channels close.
■ Potassium flows out rapidly.

Phase 4: **Resting phase**
■ Active transport through the sodium-potassium pump begins restoring potassium to the inside of the cell and sodium to the outside.
■ The cell membrane becomes impermeable to sodium.
■ Potassium may move out of the cell.

Cardiac output

Cardiac output refers to the amount of blood the heart pumps in 1 minute. To determine cardiac output, multiply the heart rate by the stroke volume (the amount of blood ejected with each heartbeat). Stroke volume depends on three factors:

Preload is the stretching of muscle fibers in the ventricles as the ventricles fill with blood. Think of preload as a balloon stretching as air is blown into it. The more air being blown, the greater the stretch.

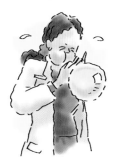

Contractility refers to the inherent ability of the myocardium to contract normally. Contractility is influenced by preload. The greater the stretch, the more forceful the contraction — or, the more air in the balloon, the greater the stretch, and the farther the balloon will fly when the air is allowed to expel.

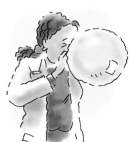

Afterload refers to the pressure that the ventricular muscles must generate to overcome the higher pressure in the aorta to get the blood out of the heart. Resistance is the knot on the end of the balloon, which the balloon has to work against to get the air out.

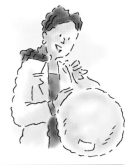

Pulling it together

When a muscle cell is in the resting state, tropomyosin and troponin (a cardiac-specific protein) inhibit contractility by preventing actin-myosin binding.

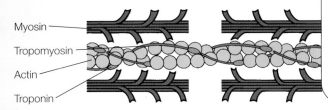

Myosin

Tropomyosin

Actin

Troponin

Electrical stimulation causes calcium release. Calcium binds to troponin, changing the configuration of tropomyosin and exposing actin-binding sites. Myosin and actin bind, creating cross-bridges, and the muscle contracts.

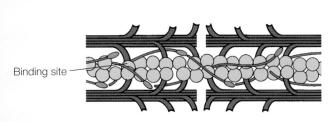

Binding site

> Wonder how the muscle contracts? Electrical stimulation causes troponin to expose actin-binding sites, which allows cardiac muscle contraction to occur.

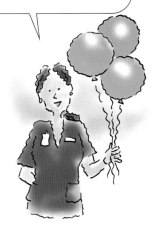

Arteriovenous circulation

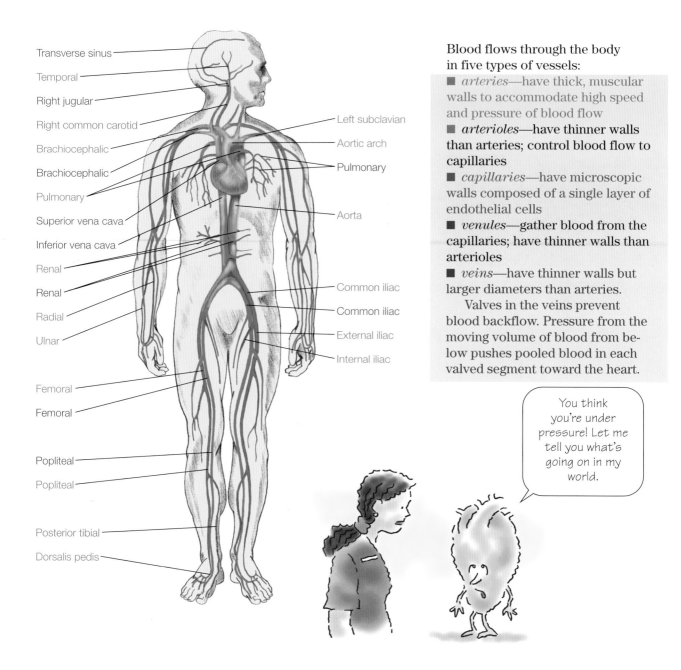

Transverse sinus

Temporal

Right jugular

Right common carotid

Brachiocephalic

Brachiocephalic

Pulmonary

Superior vena cava

Inferior vena cava

Renal

Renal

Radial

Ulnar

Femoral

Femoral

Popliteal

Popliteal

Posterior tibial

Dorsalis pedis

Left subclavian

Aortic arch

Pulmonary

Aorta

Common iliac

Common iliac

External iliac

Internal iliac

Blood flows through the body in five types of vessels:

■ *arteries*—have thick, muscular walls to accommodate high speed and pressure of blood flow

■ *arterioles*—have thinner walls than arteries; control blood flow to capillaries

■ *capillaries*—have microscopic walls composed of a single layer of endothelial cells

■ *venules*—gather blood from the capillaries; have thinner walls than arterioles

■ *veins*—have thinner walls but larger diameters than arteries.

Valves in the veins prevent blood backflow. Pressure from the moving volume of blood from below pushes pooled blood in each valved segment toward the heart.

You think you're under pressure! Let me tell you what's going on in my world.

Three methods of circulation carry blood throughout the body: pulmonary, systemic, and coronary.

Inside scoop
Blood circulation

4 …and returns to the heart.

1 Blood leaves the heart…

3 …exchanges nutrients and gases at the capillary level…

2 …reaches a body structure…

Specialized circulatory systems

The circulatory system involves more than the circulation of blood out of the heart. The heart muscle itself—as well as the liver—must receive a steady supply of oxygenated blood.

Circulation to the heart muscle

The heart relies on the coronary arteries and their branches for its supply of oxygenated blood. It also depends on the cardiac veins to remove oxygen-depleted blood.

During diastole, blood flows out of the heart and into the coronary arteries. The right coronary artery supplies blood to the right atrium, part of the left atrium, most of the right ventricle, and the inferior part of the left ventricle. The left coronary artery, which splits into the anterior descending and circumflex arteries, supplies blood to the left atrium, most of the left ventricle, and most of the interventricular septum.

The cardiac veins lie superficial to the arteries. The largest vein, the coronary sinus, opens into the right atrium. Most of the major cardiac veins empty into the coronary sinus; the anterior cardiac veins, however, empty into the right atrium.

Inside scoop
Coronary arteries

Anterior view

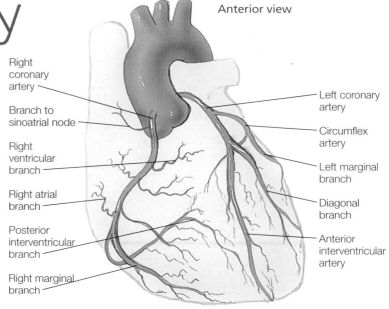

Right coronary artery
Branch to sinoatrial node
Right ventricular branch
Right atrial branch
Posterior interventricular branch
Right marginal branch

Left coronary artery
Circumflex artery
Left marginal branch
Diagonal branch
Anterior interventricular artery

Coronary veins

Posterior view

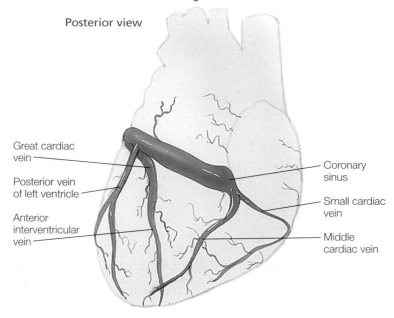

Great cardiac vein
Posterior vein of left ventricle
Anterior interventricular vein

Coronary sinus
Small cardiac vein
Middle cardiac vein

Circulation to the liver

Seventy-five percent of the blood in the liver comes from the portal vein that drains the GI tract. This blood is full of nutrients. The other 25% is oxygenated blood coming from the hepatic artery.

Capillary beds form the sinusoids of the liver, where hepatocytes filter and store nutrients and toxins. The sinusoids empty into the hepatic vein for venous return to the heart.

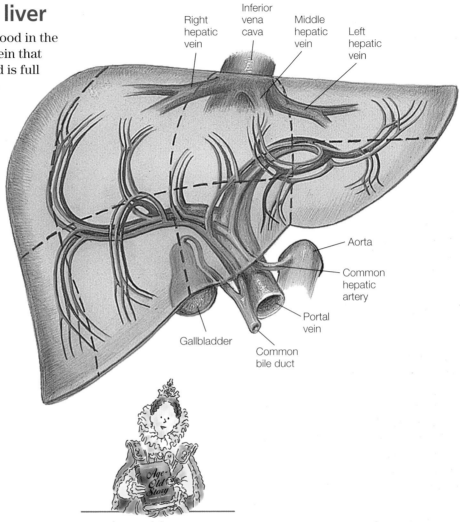

Right hepatic vein

Inferior vena cava

Middle hepatic vein

Left hepatic vein

Aorta

Common hepatic artery

Portal vein

Gallbladder

Common bile duct

Age-old story

Age-related cardiovascular changes

The heart

■ Heart becomes slightly smaller.
■ Contractile strength declines, making the heart less efficient.
■ Resting cardiac output diminishes 30% to 35% by age 70.
■ The aorta becomes more rigid, causing systolic blood pressure to rise disproportionately higher than the diastolic pressure, resulting in a widened pulse pressure.

■ Between ages 30 and 80, the left ventricular wall grows 25% thicker from its increased efforts to pump blood.
■ Heart valves become thicker from fibrotic and sclerotic changes. This can prevent the valves from closing completely, causing systolic murmurs.

Circulatory system

■ Veins dilate and stretch with age.
■ Coronary artery blood flow drops 35% between ages 20 and 60.

VISION QUEST

Able to label?

Label the heart chambers and heart valves indicated on this illustration.

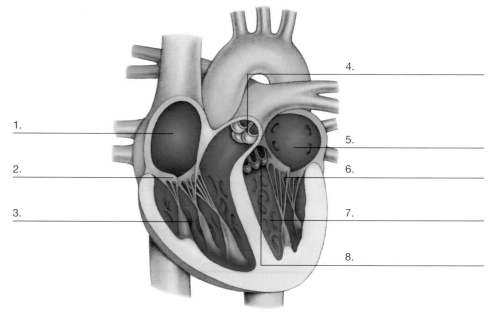

1. _____
2. _____
3. _____
4. _____
5. _____
6. _____
7. _____
8. _____

My word!

Unscramble the names of the five vessel types in the circulatory system. Then use the circled letters to answer the question posed.

Question: Which node is the heart's primary pacemaker?

1. elvesun   _ _ O _ O _ _

2. areelsriot   O _ O _ _ _ O _ _

3. siven   _ _ O _ _

4. isacalliper   _ O _ _ _ _ _ O _ _

5. eatersir   _ O _ _ _ _ O

Answer: _ _ _ _ _ _ _ _ _ _ _

10 Hematologic system

Hematology basics 108
Blood components 109
Blood clotting 112
Blood groups 115
Vision quest 116

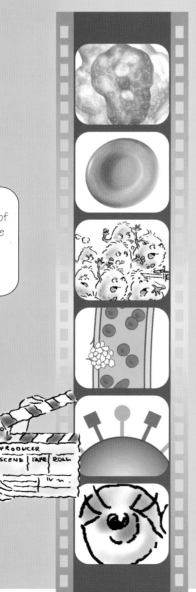

Here we go, the "lifeblood" of our story...the hematologic system, take one!

PRODUCER SCENE TAKE ROLL

Hematology basics

The hematologic system consists of the blood and bone marrow. Blood delivers oxygen and nutrients to all tissues, removes wastes, and transports gases, blood cells, immune cells, and hormones throughout the body.

The development of blood cells

The hematologic system manufactures new blood cells through a process called *hematopoiesis*.

Stem cell (hemocytoblast)

1 Multipotential stem cells in bone marrow give rise to…
2 …five distinct types of unipotential stem cells.
3 Unipotential stem cells differentiate into the various types of blood cells.

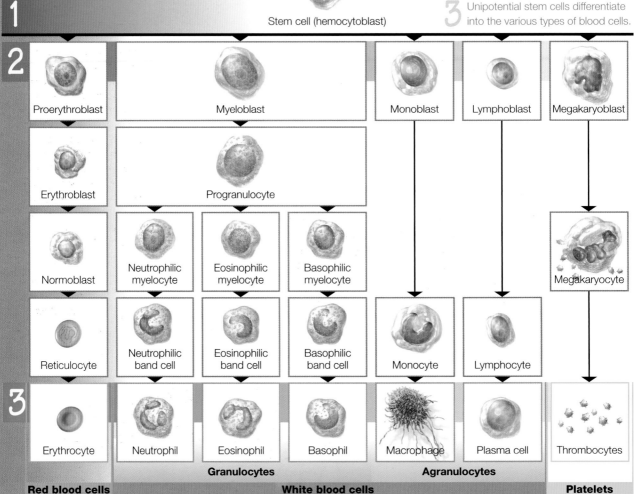

Red blood cells	Granulocytes			Agranulocytes		Platelets
Proerythroblast	Myeloblast			Monoblast	Lymphoblast	Megakaryoblast
Erythroblast	Progranulocyte					
Normoblast	Neutrophilic myelocyte	Eosinophilic myelocyte	Basophilic myelocyte			Megakaryocyte
Reticulocyte	Neutrophilic band cell	Eosinophilic band cell	Basophilic band cell	Monocyte	Lymphocyte	
Erythrocyte	Neutrophil	Eosinophil	Basophil	Macrophage	Plasma cell	Thrombocytes

Red blood cells — **Granulocytes** / **Agranulocytes** / **White blood cells** — **Platelets**

Blood components

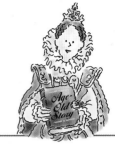

Blood consists of various formed elements, or blood cells, suspended in a fluid called *plasma*. Formed elements in the blood include:

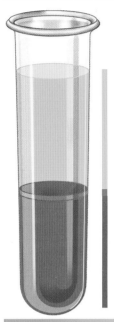

■ Plasma (55%)

■ White blood cells (WBCs) and platelets (< 1%)

■ Red blood cells (RBCs) (45%)

> RBCs and platelets function entirely within blood vessels, whereas WBCs act mainly in the tissues outside blood vessels.

Age-old story

Age-related hematologic changes

As a person ages, fatty bone marrow replaces some of the body's active blood-forming marrow—first in the long bones and later in the flat bones. The altered bone marrow can't increase erythrocyte production as readily in response to such stimuli as hormones, anoxia, hemorrhage, and hemolysis. Vitamin B_{12} absorption may also diminish with age, resulting in reduced erythrocyte mass and decreased hemoglobin levels and hematocrit.

Red blood cells

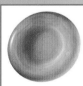

RBCs, or erythrocytes, transport oxygen and carbon dioxide to and from body tissues. They contain hemoglobin, the oxygen-carrying substance that gives blood its red color. The RBC surface carries antigens, which determine a person's blood group, or blood type.

> RBCs have an average life span of 120 days.

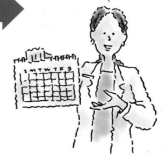

RBC timeline

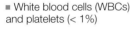

Bone marrow releases RBCs into circulation in immature form as reticulocytes.	The reticulocytes mature into RBCs in about 1 day.	The spleen isolates old, worn-out RBCs and removes them from circulation.	When RBC depletion occurs (for example, with hemorrhage) the bone marrow increases reticulocyte production to maintain the normal RBC count.

White blood cells

WBCs, or leukocytes, protect the body against harmful bacteria and infection. Most WBCs are produced in the red bone marrow from a precursor stem cell called a *hemocytoblast*. WBCs are classified as *granulocytes* or *agranulocytes*.

Granulocytes (Contain a single multilobular nucleus and granules in the cytoplasm)			Agranulocytes (Lack specific cytoplasmic granules and have a nucleus without lobes)	
Neutrophils	*Eosinophils*	*Basophils*	*Monocytes*	*Lymphocytes*

■ Most numerous, accounting for 50% to 75% of circulating WBCs ■ Engulf, ingest, and digest foreign materials (phagocytosis) ■ Worn-out neutrophils form the main component of pus	■ Account for 0.3% to 7% of circulating WBCs ■ Migrate from the bloodstream as a response to an allergic reaction ■ Defend against parasites and fight lung and skin infections	■ Constitute fewer than 2% of circulating WBCs ■ Possess little or no phagocytic ability ■ May release heparin and histamine into blood and participate in delayed allergic reactions	■ Largest of the WBCs ■ Constitute 1% to 9% of WBCs in circulation ■ Devour invading organisms by phagocytosis ■ Migrate to tissue where they develop into macrophages, which participate in immunity ▼ 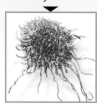	■ Smallest of the WBCs ■ Constitute 20% to 43% of WBCs ■ Derive from stem cells in the bone marrow ■ Consist of two types: – T lymphocytes, which directly attack an infected cell – B lymphocytes, which produce antibodies against specific antigens

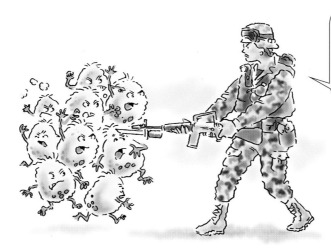

WBCs are like soldiers fighting off the enemy. Each type of WBC fights a different enemy.

On the front line

Granulocytes, with "platoons" of basophils, neutrophils, and eosinophils, are the first forces "marshaled" against invading foreign organisms.

Basophils spit histamine at inflammatory and immune stimuli.

Neutrophils eat foreign bodies.

Eosinophils eat antigens and antibodies.

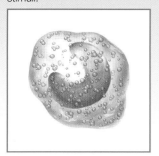

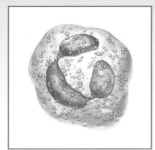

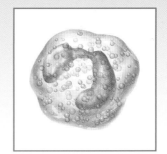

In the trenches

Agranulocytes, with "platoons" of lymphocytes and monocytes, may roam freely on "patrol" when inflammation is reported, but they mainly "dig in" at structures that filter large amounts of fluid (such as the liver) and defend against invaders.

Lymphocytes eat the enemy, or produce antibodies.

Monocytes eat bacteria, cellular debris, and necrotic tissue.

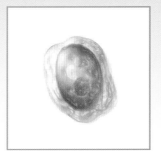

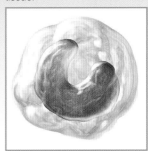

Platelets

Platelets, or *thrombocytes*, are small, colorless, disk-shaped cytoplasmic fragments split from cells in bone marrow called *megakaryocytes*. These fragments, which have a life span of approximately 10 days, perform three vital functions:

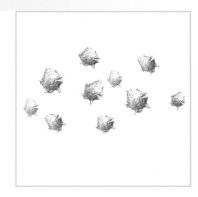

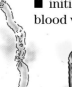

- initiate contraction of damaged blood vessels to minimize blood loss
- provide materials (along with plasma) that accelerate blood coagulation
- form hemostatic plugs in injured blood vessels.

Blood clotting

Hemostasis is the complex process by which platelets, plasma, and coagulation factors interact to control bleeding.

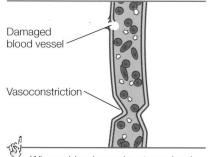

Damaged blood vessel

Vasoconstriction

When a blood vessel ruptures, local *vasoconstriction* (decrease in the caliber of blood vessels) occurs to decrease blood flow to the area.

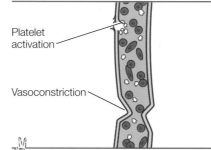

Platelet activation

Vasoconstriction

Platelets and clotting factors become activated when exposed to the collagen layer of the damaged blood vessel.

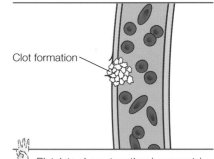

Clot formation

Platelets clump together (*aggregate*) by binding to the collagen, forming a loose platelet plug.

Aggregation provides a temporary seal and a site for clotting to take place.

However, formation of a more stable clot requires initiation of the complex clotting mechanisms known as the *intrinsic cascade system*.

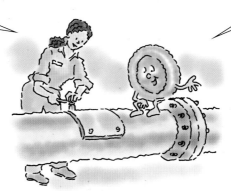

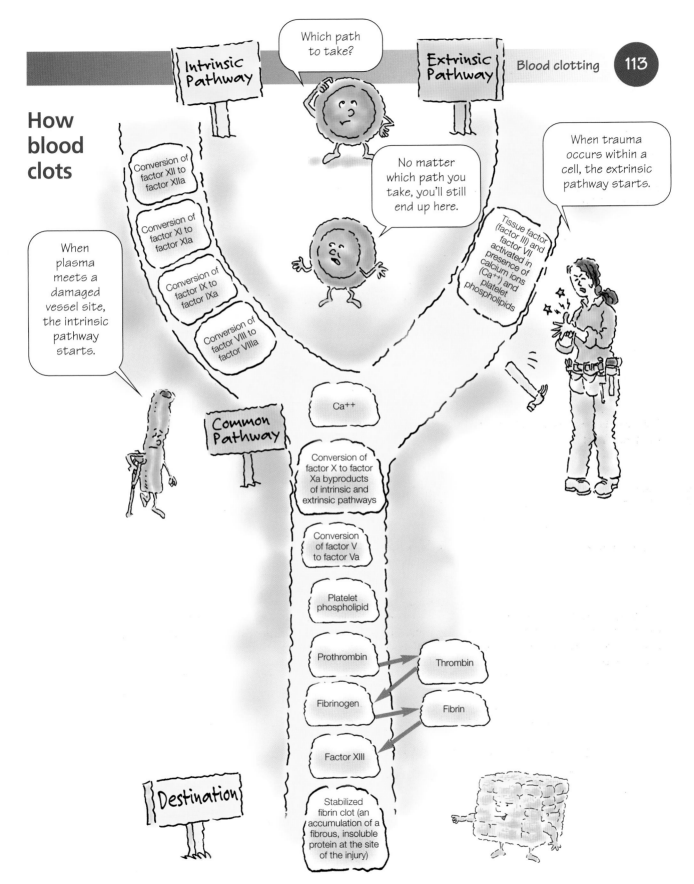

Coagulation factors

Coagulation factors are:

■ made up of plasma proteins—except for factor IV (calcium), which is a mineral, and factor III (thromboplastin), which is a lipoprotein released from tissue
■ produced in the liver
■ activated in a chain reaction, with each one in turn activating the next factor in the chain.

> Coagulation factors are named according to a system of Roman numerals that relate to their order of discovery— not their order in a reaction.

Factor I
■ Fibrinogen
■ Converts to fibrin when blood clots

Factor II
■ Prothrombin
■ Inactive precursor to thrombin

Factor III
■ Tissue thromboplastin
■ Converts prothrombin to thrombin as blood starts to clot

Factor IV
■ Consists of calcium ions
■ Required throughout the entire clotting sequence

Factor V
■ Labile factor (proaccelerin)
■ Functions during the combined pathway phase of the coagulation system

Factor VII
■ Also known as serum prothrombin conversion accelerator or stable factor (proconvertin)
■ Activated by Factor III in the extrinsic system

Factor VIII
■ Antihemophilic factor
■ Required during the intrinsic phase of the coagulation system.

Factor IX
■ Plasma thromboplastin component
■ Required in the intrinsic phase of the coagulation system

Factor X
■ Stuart factor (Stuart-Prower factor)
■ Required in the combined pathway of the coagulation system

Factor XI
■ Plasma thromboplastin antecedent
■ Required in the intrinsic system

Factor XII
■ Hageman factor
■ Required in the intrinsic system

Factor XIII
■ Fibrin-stabilizing factor
■ Required to stabilize fibrin strands in the combined pathway phase of the coagulation system

Blood groups

Blood groups are determined by the presence or absence of genetically determined antigens or agglutinogens (glycoproteins) on the surface of RBCs. (A, B, and Rh are the most clinically significant blood antigens.) Plasma may contain *antibodies* that interact with the antigens on other RBC types, causing the cells to *agglutinate*, or clump together.

> Plasma can't contain antibodies to its own cell antigen or it would destroy itself. As you can see here, type A blood has A antigen but no A antibodies; however, it does have B antibodies.

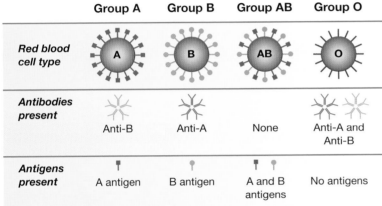

	Group A	Group B	Group AB	Group O
Red blood cell type	A	B	AB	O
Antibodies present	Anti-B	Anti-A	None	Anti-A and Anti-B
Antigens present	A antigen	B antigen	A and B antigens	No antigens

Rh typing

Rh typing determines whether the Rh antigen (called the *Rh factor*) is present or absent in the blood:

■ If RBCs have the Rh antigen, the blood is Rh-positive.

■ If RBCs don't have the Rh antigen, it's Rh-negative.

When a person who is Rh-negative becomes sensitized to the Rh antigen—such as following a transfusion of Rh-positive blood or when an Rh-negative female carries an Rh-positive fetus—anti-Rh antibodies can develop.

> If blood has both A and Rh antigens, it's called *A positive* (A⁺). If blood has B antigens but not the Rh antigen, it's called *B negative* (B⁻).

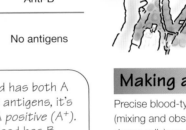

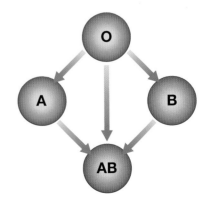

Making a match

Precise blood-typing and crossmatching (mixing and observing for agglutination of donor cells) are essential, especially for blood transfusions. A donor's blood must be compatible with a recipient's or the result can be fatal. These blood groups are compatible:

■ type A with type A or O

■ type B with type B or O

■ type AB with type A, B, AB, or O

■ type O with type O only.

VISION QUEST

Matchmaker

Match each type of blood component with its main function.

1. Erythrocytes
2. Leukocytes
3. Platelets
4. Stem cells

A. Perform a key role in blood clotting
B. Protect the body against harmful bacteria
C. Transport oxygen and carbon dioxide to and from body tissues
D. Give rise to the cells that differentiate into the various types of blood cells

Show and tell

Describe the steps in blood clot formation illustrated here.

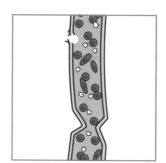

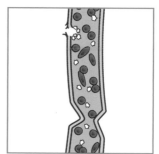

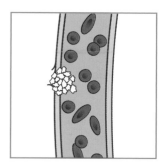

1. _____

_____
_____
_____
_____
_____
_____
_____
_____
_____
_____

2. _____

_____
_____
_____
_____
_____
_____
_____
_____
_____
_____

3. _____

_____
_____
_____
_____
_____
_____
_____
_____
_____
_____

11
Immune system

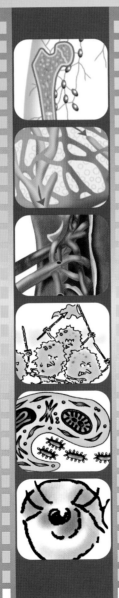

■ Immune system
  structures 118
■ Functions of the
  immune system 128
■ Vision quest 132

This chapter has all the makings of a great action-adventure! I can picture it now: the immune system nobly defending the body against invasion by harmful organisms and chemical toxins!

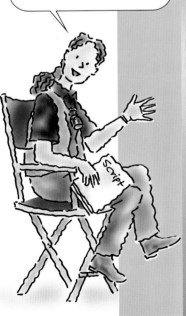

Immune system structures

Organs and tissues of the immune system are referred to as "lymphoid" because they're all involved with the growth, development, and dissemination of lymphocytes, one type of white blood cell (WBC).

The immune system has three major divisions:

1 Central lymphoid organs and tissues

2 Peripheral lymphoid organs and tissues

3 Accessory lymphoid organs and tissues

Although the immune system and blood are distinct entities, each shares a common origin in the bone marrow. What's more, the immune system uses the bloodstream to transport its "troops" to the site of an invasion.

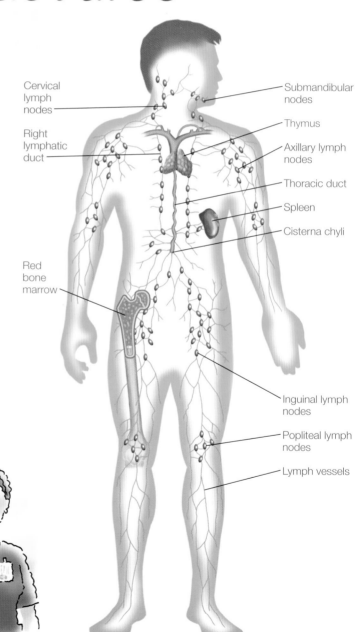

Cervical lymph nodes

Right lymphatic duct

Red bone marrow

Submandibular nodes

Thymus

Axillary lymph nodes

Thoracic duct

Spleen

Cisterna chyli

Inguinal lymph nodes

Popliteal lymph nodes

Lymph vessels

Central lymphoid organs and tissues

The bone marrow and thymus play distinctive roles in the development of B cells and T cells, two major types of lymphocytes.

Cells of the immune system and the blood both develop from stem cells in a process called hematopoiesis.

The stem cells found in bone marrow are multipotential, meaning they're capable of taking many forms and can develop into any of several different cell types.

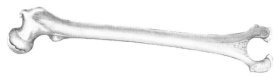

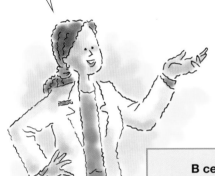

Bone marrow

Lymphocytes

Phagocytes
(ingest microorganisms)

B cells
(mature in bone marrow)

T cells
(travel to thymus and mature there)

Produce antibodies (molecules that attack pathogens or direct other cells to attack them)

Thymus

■ Two-lobed mass of lymphoid tissue located over the base of the heart in the mediastinum in fetuses and infants

■ Helps form T lymphocytes for several months after birth

■ Gradually atrophies until only a remnant persists in adults

■ "Trains" T cells to recognize other cells from the same body (self cells) and distinguish them from all other cells (nonself cells)

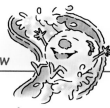

Go with the flow

B-cell formation

The formation of B cells consists of two stages. The first stage occurs shortly after birth; the second stage occurs when an immature B cell encounters its specific antigen.

Stage 1

STEM CELLS

Shortly before and after birth, stem cells develop into:

IMMATURE B CELLS

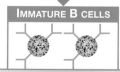

These are small lymphocytes with antibody molecules in their cytoplasmic membranes. Immature B cells migrate to the lymph nodes, liver, and spleen.

Stage 2   If immature B cells contact a specific antigen, the antigen binds to the antibody on the surface of the immature B cells, changing them into:

ACTIVATED B CELLS

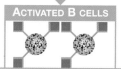

These cells divide rapidly and repeatedly to form clones of:

MEMORY CELLS

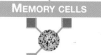

PLASMA CELLS

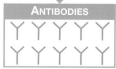

Memory cells are stored in lymph nodes. Subsequent exposure to the specific antigen changes the memory cells into plasma cells.

Plasma cells secrete antibodies into the blood.

ANTIBODIES

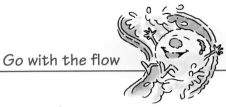

Go with the flow

T-cell formation

T cells are lymphocytes that have undergone their first stage of development in the thymus. The second stage of development occurs when they contact an antigen.

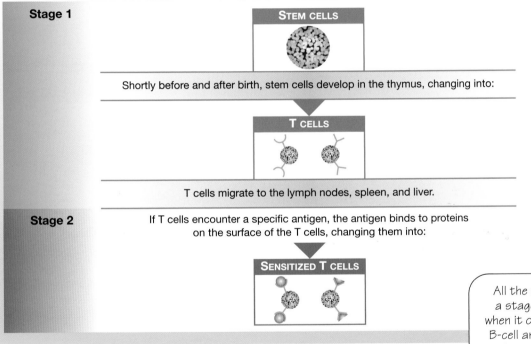

Stage 1

STEM CELLS

Shortly before and after birth, stem cells develop in the thymus, changing into:

T CELLS

T cells migrate to the lymph nodes, spleen, and liver.

Stage 2

If T cells encounter a specific antigen, the antigen binds to proteins on the surface of the T cells, changing them into:

SENSITIZED T CELLS

All the world's a stage, even when it comes to B-cell and T-cell formation.

Peripheral lymphoid organs and tissues

Lymph nodes

The lymph nodes are small, oval-shaped structures located along a network of lymph channels. Most abundant in the head, neck, axillae, abdomen, pelvis, and groin, they help remove and destroy antigens (substances capable of triggering an immune response) that circulate in the blood and lymph.

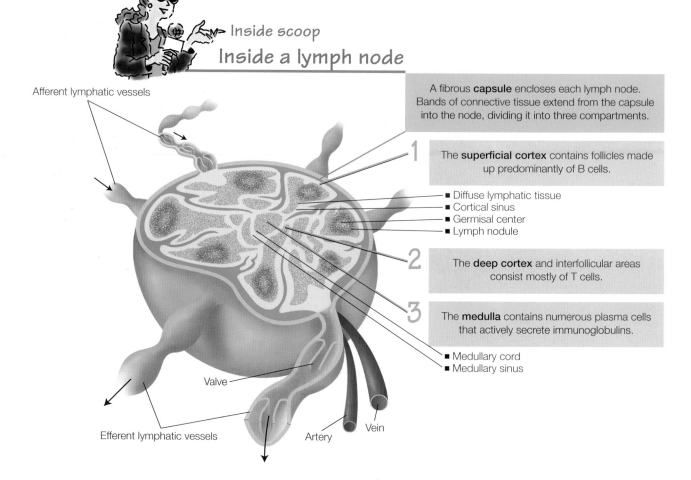

Inside scoop

Inside a lymph node

Afferent lymphatic vessels

A fibrous **capsule** encloses each lymph node. Bands of connective tissue extend from the capsule into the node, dividing it into three compartments.

1 The **superficial cortex** contains follicles made up predominantly of B cells.

- Diffuse lymphatic tissue
- Cortical sinus
- Germisal center
- Lymph nodule

2 The **deep cortex** and interfollicular areas consist mostly of T cells.

3 The **medulla** contains numerous plasma cells that actively secrete immunoglobulins.

- Medullary cord
- Medullary sinus

Valve

Efferent lymphatic vessels

Artery

Vein

Lymph and lymphatic vessels

Lymph is a clear fluid that bathes the body tissues, moving through the intracellular spaces via the lymphatic vessels.

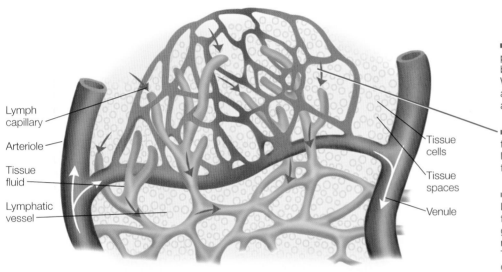

Lymph capillary

Arteriole

Tissue fluid

Lymphatic vessel

Tissue cells

Tissue spaces

Venule

■ Lymph contains a liquid portion, which resembles blood plasma, as well as WBCs (mostly lymphocytes and macrophages) and antigens.

■ Collected from body tissues, lymph seeps into lymphatic vessels across the vessels' thin walls.

■ Because numerous nodes line the lymphatic channels that drain a particular region, lymph travels through more than one lymph node. This arrangement prevents organisms that enter peripheral areas from migrating unchallenged to central areas.

The path of lymph

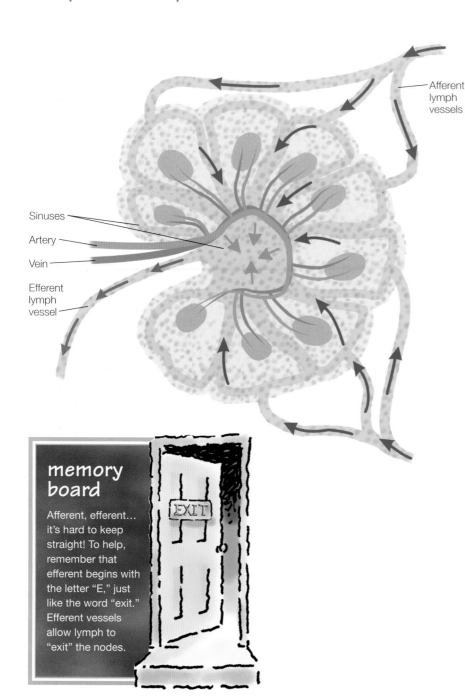

Afferent lymph vessels

Sinuses

Artery

Vein

Efferent lymph vessel

Afferent lymphatic vessels carry lymph into the subcapsular sinus (or cavity) of the lymph node.

Lymph then flows through cortical sinuses and smaller radial medullary sinuses.

Phagocytic cells in the deep cortex and medullary sinuses attack antigens carried in lymph.

Cleansed lymph leaves the node through efferent lymphatic vessels at the hilum (a depression at the exit or entrance of the node).

memory board

Afferent, efferent… it's hard to keep straight! To help, remember that efferent begins with the letter "E," just like the word "exit." Efferent vessels allow lymph to "exit" the nodes.

EXIT

Lymphatic vessels drain into lymph node chains that, in turn, empty into large lymph vessels, or trunks, that drain into the subclavian vein of the vascular system.

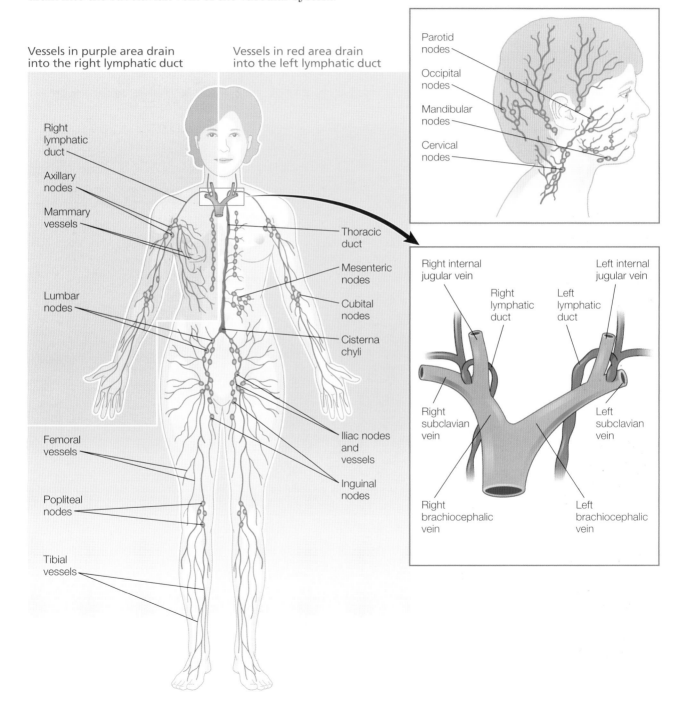

Vessels in purple area drain into the right lymphatic duct

Vessels in red area drain into the left lymphatic duct

Right lymphatic duct

Axillary nodes

Mammary vessels

Lumbar nodes

Femoral vessels

Popliteal nodes

Tibial vessels

Thoracic duct

Mesenteric nodes

Cubital nodes

Cisterna chyli

Iliac nodes and vessels

Inguinal nodes

Parotid nodes

Occipital nodes

Mandibular nodes

Cervical nodes

Right internal jugular vein

Right lymphatic duct

Left lymphatic duct

Left internal jugular vein

Right subclavian vein

Left subclavian vein

Right brachiocephalic vein

Left brachiocephalic vein

Spleen

The spleen is a dark red, oval structure that's approximately the size of a fist. The interior, called the *splenic pulp*, contains white and red pulp.

White pulp
- Contains compact masses of lymphocytes
- Surrounds branches of the splenic artery

Red pulp
- Consists of a network of blood-filled sinusoids
- Supported by a framework of reticular fibers and mononuclear phagocytes, along with some lymphocytes, plasma cells, and monocytes

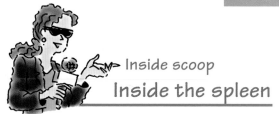

Inside scoop

Inside the spleen

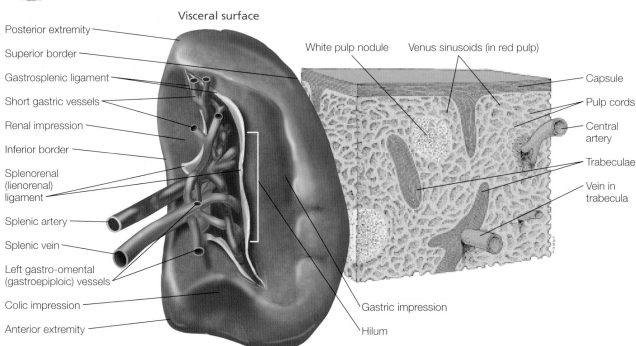

Visceral surface

- Posterior extremity
- Superior border
- Gastrosplenic ligament
- Short gastric vessels
- Renal impression
- Inferior border
- Splenorenal (lienorenal) ligament
- Splenic artery
- Splenic vein
- Left gastro-omental (gastroepiploic) vessels
- Colic impression
- Anterior extremity

- White pulp nodule
- Venus sinusoids (in red pulp)
- Capsule
- Pulp cords
- Central artery
- Trabeculae
- Vein in trabecula

- Gastric impression
- Hilum

The spleen's functions

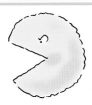

■ Engulfs and breaks down worn-out red blood cells (RBCs), causing the release of hemoglobin, which then breaks down into its components

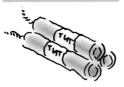

■ Retains and destroys damaged or abnormal RBCs and cells with large amounts of abnormal hemoglobin

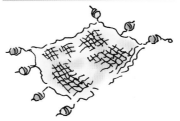

■ Filters and removes bacteria and other foreign substances that enter the bloodstream

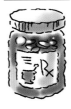

■ Initiates an immune response

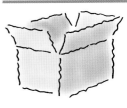

■ Stores blood and 20% to 30% of platelets

Accessory lymphoid organs and tissues

The tonsils, adenoids, appendix, and Peyer's patches remove foreign debris in much the same way lymph nodes do. They're located in food and air passages—areas where microbial access is likely to occur.

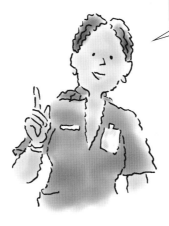

The easiest way for microbes to enter our bodies is through the food we eat and the air we breathe. That's why food and air passages contain accessory lymphoid organs and tissues.

Functions of the immune system

The immune system is designed to recognize, respond to, and eliminate antigens, including bacteria, fungi, viruses, and parasites. It also preserves the body's internal environment by scavenging dead or damaged cells and patrolling for antigens. To perform these functions efficiently, the immune system uses three basic strategies.

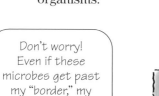

Protective surface phenomena

Strategically placed physical, chemical, and mechanical barriers work to prevent the entry of potentially harmful organisms.

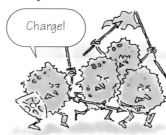

Charge!

First line of defense

- Intact and healing skin and mucous membranes (prevent attachment of microorganisms)
- Normal cell turnover and low pH (further impede bacterial colonization)

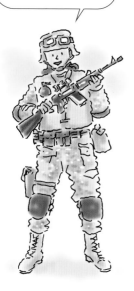

Don't worry! Even if these microbes get past my "border," my "interior troops" are on alert.

Second line of defense

Organ system		Immune function
Nose		▪ Nasal hairs and turbulent airflow filter foreign materials. ▪ Immunoglobulin in nasal secretions discourages microbe adherence.
Respiratory tract		▪ Mucous lining in the respiratory tract traps microorganisms. ▪ Cilia lining the upper respiratory tract sweep dust particles and bacteria toward the mouth, preventing them from entering the lower respiratory tract.
GI tract		▪ Saliva, swallowing, peristalsis, and defecation mechanically remove bacteria. ▪ Low pH of gastric secretions is *bactericidal* (bacteria-killing), rendering the stomach virtually free from live bacteria. ▪ Resident bacteria in the rest of the GI system prevent other microorganisms from permanently making a home.
Urinary tract		▪ Urine flow, low urine pH, immunoglobulin and, in men, the bactericidal effects of prostatic fluid work together to impede bacterial colonization. ▪ A series of sphincters inhibits bacterial migration.

General host defenses

When an antigen does penetrate the skin or mucous membrane, the immune system launches nonspecific cellular responses in an effort to identify and remove the invader.

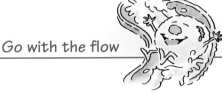

Go with the flow

The inflammatory response

Microorganisms invade damaged tissue.

Basophils release heparin, and histamine and kinin production occurs.

Vasodilation occurs along with increased capillary permeability.

Blood flow increases to the affected tissue, and fluid collects within it.

Neutrophils flock to the invasion site to engulf and destroy microorganisms.

Tissue repair occurs.

Specific immune responses

Invasion of a foreign substance can trigger two types of immune responses—antibody-mediated (humoral) and cell-mediated immunity:

■ In *antibody-mediated* immunity, antigens stimulate B cells to differentiate into plasma cells and produce circulating antibodies that disable bacteria and viruses before they can enter host cells.

■ In *cell-mediated* immunity, T cells move directly to attack invaders. Three T-cell subgroups trigger the response to infection. Helper T cells spur B cells to manufacture antibodies. Effector T cells kill antigens and produce lymphokines (proteins that induce inflammatory response and mediate the delayed hypersensitivity reaction). Suppressor T cells regulate T and B types of immune responses.

In cell-mediated immunity, I'm on guard, ready to attack invaders.

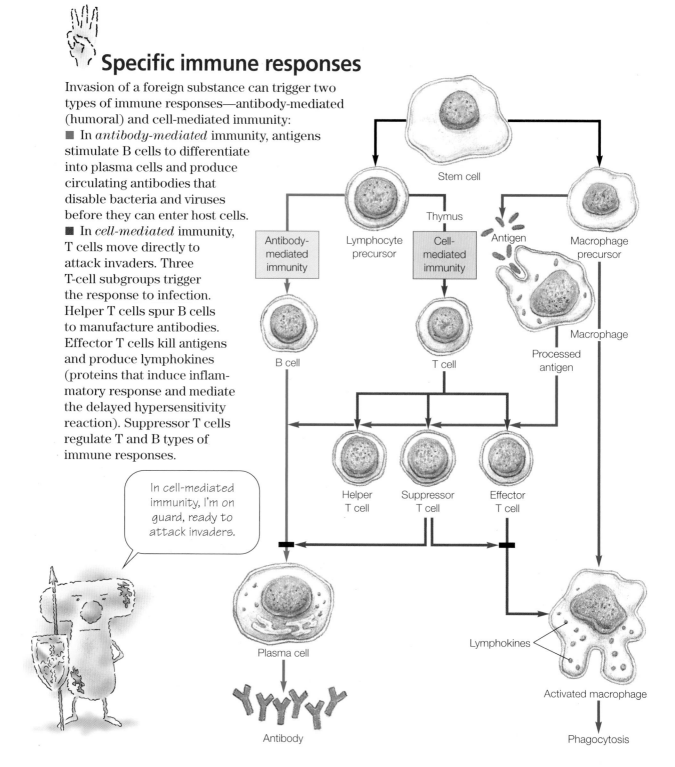

How macrophages accomplish phagocytosis

Microorganisms and other antigens that invade the skin and mucous membranes are removed by *phagocytosis,* a defense mechanism carried out by macrophages (mononuclear leukocytes) and neutrophils (polymorphonuclear leukocytes). Here's how macrophages accomplish phagocytosis.

1 Chemotaxis

Chemotactic factors attract macrophages to the antigen site.

Macrophage

Microorganism

Chemotactic factors

2 Opsonization

Antibody (immunoglobulin G) or complement fragment coats the microorganism, enhancing macrophage binding to the antigen, now called an *opsinogen.*

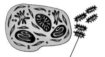
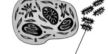

Opsonized microorganism

3 Ingestion

The macrophage extends its membrane around the opsonized microorgan-ism, engulfing it within a vacuole *(phagosome).*

Developing phagosome

4 Digestion

As the phagosome shifts away from the cell periph-ery, it merges with lyso-somes, forming a *phago-lysosome,* where antigen destruction occurs.

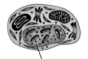

Phagolysosome

5 Release

When digestion is com-plete, the macrophage expels digestive debris, including lysosomes, prostaglandins, comple-ment components, and interferon, which continue to mediate the immune response.

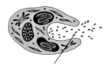

Digestive debris

Complement system

Indispensable to the humoral immune response, the complement system consists of about 25 enzymes that "complement" the work of antibodies by aiding phagocytosis or destroying bacteria cells (through puncture of their cell membranes).

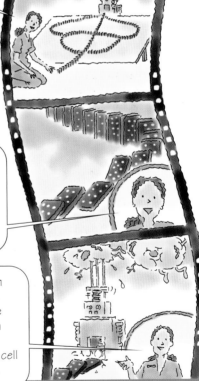

Complement proteins travel in the bloodstream in an inactive form. When the first complement substance is triggered (typically by an antibody interlocked with an antigen), it sets in motion a ripple effect.

As each component is activated in turn, it acts on the next component in a sequence of carefully controlled steps called the complement cascade.

This cascade leads to the creation of the membrane attack complex. Inserted into the membrane of the target cell, this complex creates a channel through which fluids and molecules flow in and out. The target cell then swells and eventually bursts.

By-products of the complement cascade also produce:
- the inflammatory response (resulting from release of the contents of mast cells and basophils)
- stimulation and attraction of neutrophils (which participate in phagocytosis)
- coating of target cells by C3b (an inactivated fragment of the complement protein C3), making them attractive to phagocytes.

VISION QUEST

Able to label?

Identify the organs of the lymphatic system indicated in this illustration.

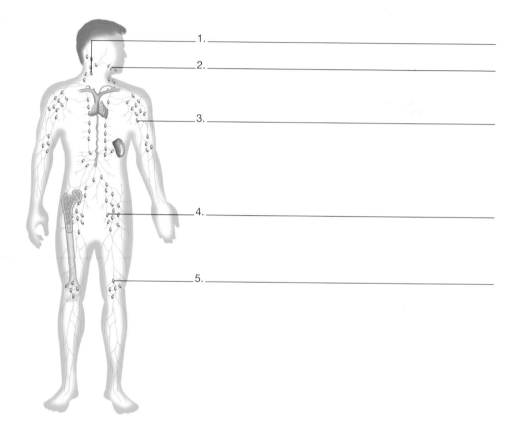

1. _____
2. _____
3. _____

4. _____

5. _____

Rebus riddle

Sound out each group of pictures and symbols to reveal a fact about the immune system.

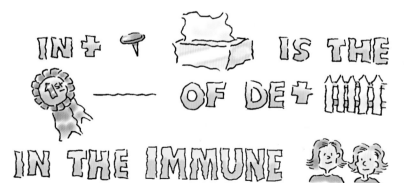

12
Respiratory system

■ Respiratory system structures 134
■ Inspiration and expiration 144
■ Vision quest 150

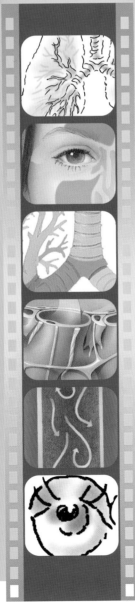

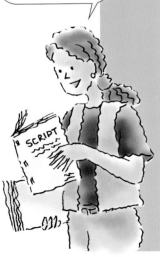

I think you'll find this chapter truly inspiring. Really...it reads like a breath of fresh air!

Respiratory system structures

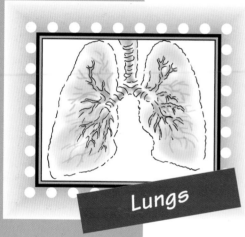

Lungs

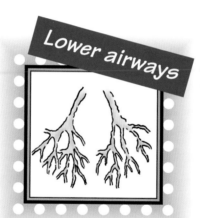

Lower airways

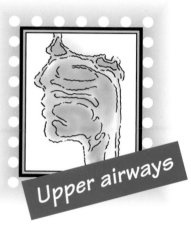

Upper airways

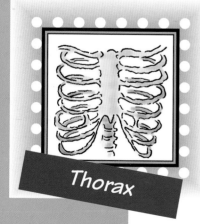

Thorax

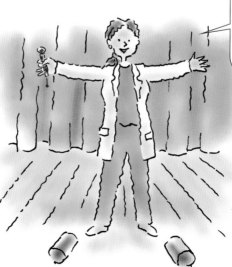

The act of breathing is a great production, requiring all these systems to work together to deliver oxygen to the bloodstream and remove excess carbon dioxide.

The structures of the upper airways—which include the nose, mouth, sinuses, laryngopharynx, and larynx—warm, filter, and humidify inhaled air.

Upper airways

Nasopharynx

- Frontal sinus
- Nasal concha
- Middle nasal concha
- Sphenoid sinus
- Internal naris
- Nasopharynx
- Inferior nasal concha

Bony structures called *conchae*, or *turbinates*, form the posterior walls of the nasal passages. The conchae warm and humidify air before it passes into the naso-pharynx. Their mucus layer also traps finer foreign particles, which the cilia carry to the pharynx to be swallowed.

Air enters the body through the nostrils (nares), where small hairs called *cilia* filter out dust and large foreign particles. Air then passes into the two nasal passages, which are separated by the septum. Cartilage forms the anterior walls of the nasal passages.

Sinuses

Four pairs of paranasal sinuses open into the internal nose:

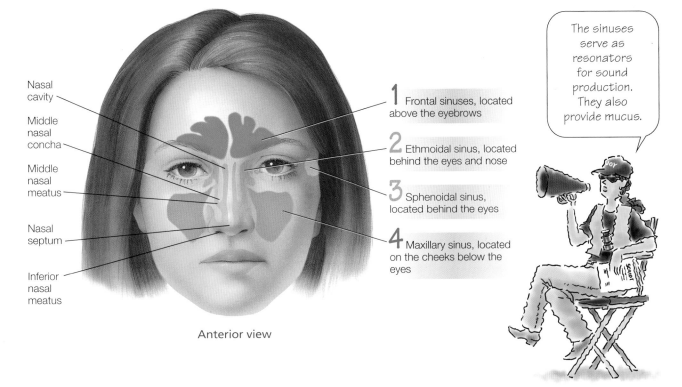

Nasal cavity

Middle nasal concha

Middle nasal meatus

Nasal septum

Inferior nasal meatus

1 Frontal sinuses, located above the eyebrows

2 Ethmoidal sinus, located behind the eyes and nose

3 Sphenoidal sinus, located behind the eyes

4 Maxillary sinus, located on the cheeks below the eyes

Anterior view

The sinuses serve as resonators for sound production. They also provide mucus.

Oropharynx and laryngopharynx

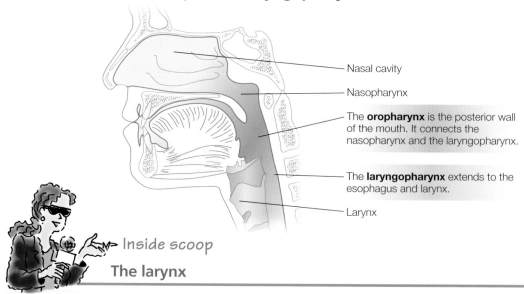

Nasal cavity

Nasopharynx

The **oropharynx** is the posterior wall of the mouth. It connects the nasopharynx and the laryngopharynx.

The **laryngopharynx** extends to the esophagus and larynx.

Larynx

Inside scoop

The larynx

The larynx houses the vocal cords. It's the transition point between the upper and lower airways. The epiglottis, a flap of tissue that closes over the top of the larynx when the patient swallows, protects the patient from aspirating food or fluid into the lower airways.

Anterior view

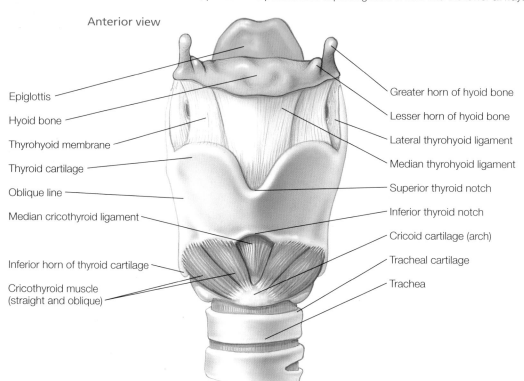

Epiglottis

Hyoid bone

Thyrohyoid membrane

Thyroid cartilage

Oblique line

Median cricothyroid ligament

Inferior horn of thyroid cartilage

Cricothyroid muscle (straight and oblique)

Greater horn of hyoid bone

Lesser horn of hyoid bone

Lateral thyrohyoid ligament

Median thyrohyoid ligament

Superior thyroid notch

Inferior thyroid notch

Cricoid cartilage (arch)

Tracheal cartilage

Trachea

Lower airways

The lower respiratory tract consists of the trachea, bronchi, and lungs.

Trachea

The **trachea** extends from the *cricoid cartilage* at the top to the *carina* (also called the *tracheal bifurcation*).

The **carina** is a ridge-shaped structure at the level of the second anterior rib, just below the aortic arch. C-shaped cartilage rings reinforce and protect the trachea to prevent it from collapsing. The primary bronchi begin at the carina.

Bronchi

The **bronchi**—along with blood vessels, nerves, and lymphatics—enter the lungs at the hilum.

The **right mainstem bronchus,** which is shorter, wider, and more vertical than the left, supplies air to the right lung.

The **left mainstem bronchus** delivers air to the left lung.

The mainstem bronchi divide into the five **lobar bronchi** (secondary bronchi). Each lobar bronchus enters a lobe in each lung.

Within its lobe, each of the lobar bronchi branches into **segmental bronchi** (tertiary bronchi).

The segments continue to branch into smaller and smaller bronchi, finally branching into **bronchioles.**

The larger bronchi consist of cartilage, smooth muscle, mucous glands, and epithelium. As the bronchi become smaller, they lose cartilage and then smooth muscle. Finally, the smallest bronchioles consist of just a single layer of epithelial cells.

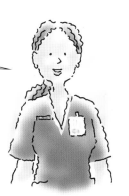

Bronchioles

Each bronchiole divides into terminal bronchioles and an acinus—the chief respiratory unit for gas exchange.

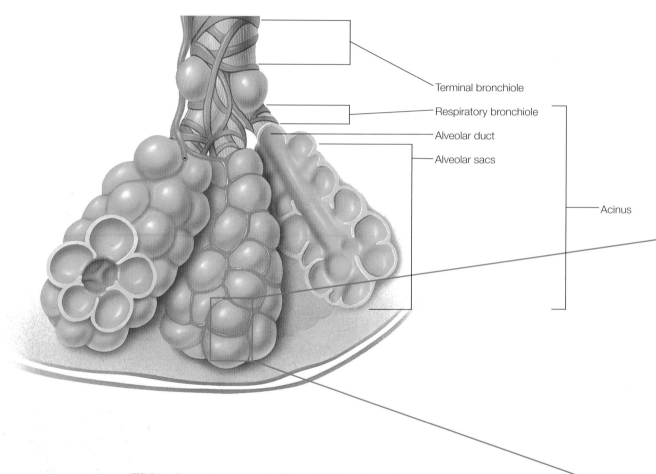

Terminal bronchiole

Respiratory bronchiole

Alveolar duct

Alveolar sacs

Acinus

Within the acinus, terminal bronchioles branch into yet smaller respiratory bronchioles. These respiratory bronchioles feed directly into alveoli at sites along their walls. The respiratory bronchioles eventually become alveolar ducts, which terminate in clusters called *alveolar sacs*.

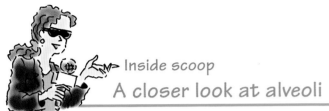

Inside scoop

A closer look at alveoli

The lungs contain millions of tiny, thin-membraned alveoli. Inside these air sacs, oxygen (O_2) from inhaled air diffuses into the blood while carbon dioxide (CO_2) diffuses from the blood into the air and is exhaled.

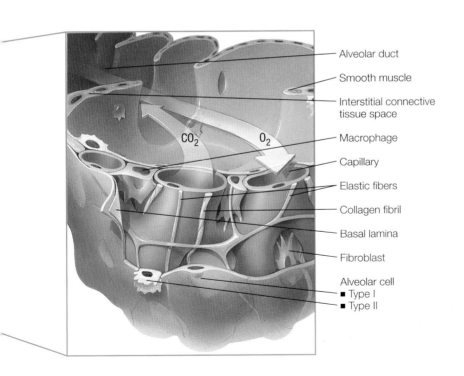

- Alveolar duct
- Smooth muscle
- Interstitial connective tissue space
- Macrophage
- Capillary
- Elastic fibers
- Collagen fibril
- Basal lamina
- Fibroblast
- Alveolar cell
  - Type I
  - Type II

CO_2 O_2

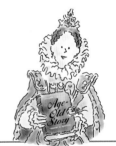

Age-old story

Insufficient surfactant

Without surfactant, surface tension can restrict alveolar expansion during inspiration and cause alveolar collapse during expiration. Surfactant is commonly lacking in preterm neonates (those born before 28 weeks' gestation) and can cause respiratory distress syndrome.

Surfactant deficiency in adults also causes alveolar collapse and adult respiratory distress syndrome.

Lungs and accessory structures

The cone-shaped lungs hang suspended in the right and left pleural cavities, straddling the heart and anchored by root and pulmonary ligaments.

Inside scoop
Lung lobes

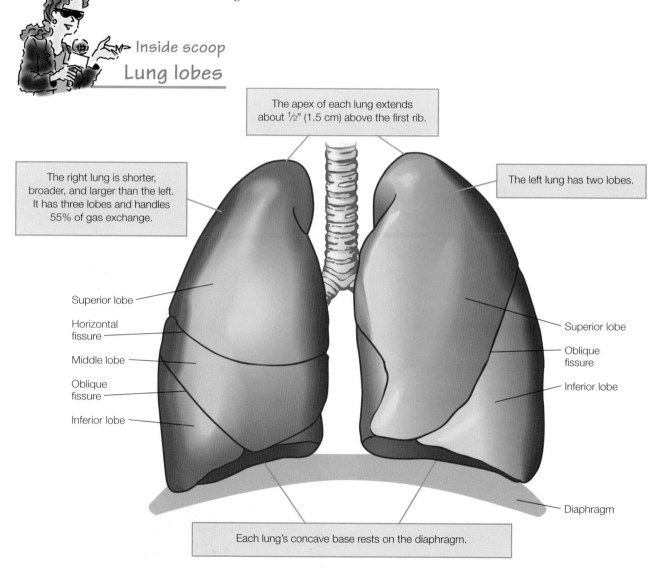

The apex of each lung extends about ½″ (1.5 cm) above the first rib.

The right lung is shorter, broader, and larger than the left. It has three lobes and handles 55% of gas exchange.

The left lung has two lobes.

Superior lobe

Horizontal fissure

Middle lobe

Oblique fissure

Inferior lobe

Superior lobe

Oblique fissure

Inferior lobe

Diaphragm

Each lung's concave base rests on the diaphragm.

Pleura and pleural cavities

The pleura—the membrane that totally encloses the lung—
is composed of a visceral layer and a parietal layer.

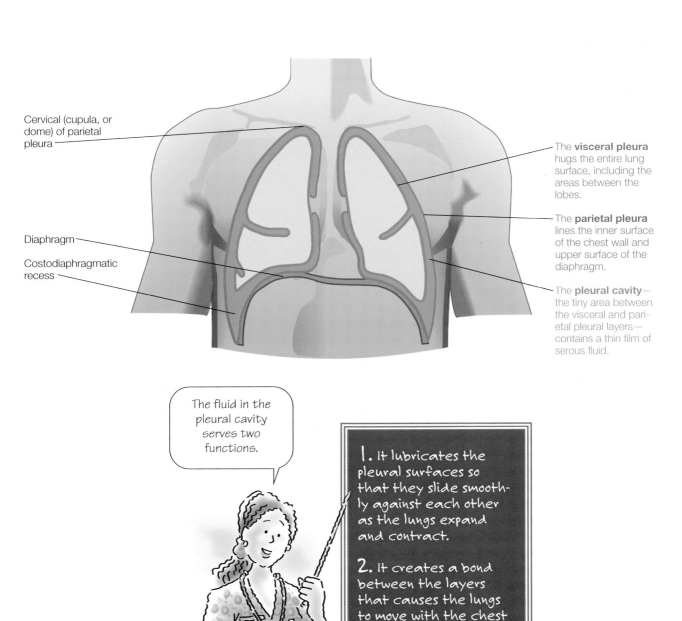

Cervical (cupula, or dome) of parietal pleura

Diaphragm

Costodiaphragmatic recess

The **visceral pleura** hugs the entire lung surface, including the areas between the lobes.

The **parietal pleura** lines the inner surface of the chest wall and upper surface of the diaphragm.

The **pleural cavity**—the tiny area between the visceral and parietal pleural layers—contains a thin film of serous fluid.

The fluid in the pleural cavity serves two functions.

1. It lubricates the pleural surfaces so that they slide smoothly against each other as the lungs expand and contract.

2. It creates a bond between the layers that causes the lungs to move with the chest wall during breathing.

Mediastinum

The space between the lungs is called the *mediastinum.* It contains the:

■ heart and pericardium
■ thoracic aorta
■ pulmonary artery and veins
■ venae cavae and azygos veins
■ thymus, lymph nodes, and vessels
■ trachea, esophagus, and thoracic duct
■ vagus, cardiac, and phrenic nerves.

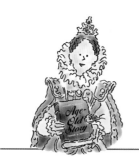

Age-old story

Age-related respiratory changes

Structural changes

■ Nose enlargement (from continued cartilage growth)
■ General atrophy of the tonsils
■ Tracheal deviations (from changes in the aging spine)
■ Increased anteroposterior chest diameter (resulting from altered calcium metabolism)
■ Calcification of costal cartilages (resulting in reduced mobility of the chest wall)
■ Kyphosis (due to osteoporosis and vertebral collapse)
■ Increased lung rigidity
■ Decreased number and dilation of alveoli
■ Reduction in respiratory fluids by 30% (heightening the risk of pulmonary infection and mucus plugs)
■ Reduction in respiratory muscle strength

Pulmonary function changes

■ Diminished ventilatory capacity
■ Decline in diffusing capacity
■ Diminished vital capacity (due to decreased inspiratory and expiratory muscle strength)
■ Decreased elastic recoil capability (resulting in an elevated residual volume)
■ Decreased ventilation of basal areas (due to closing of some airways)

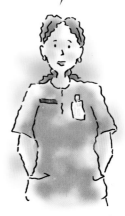

Aging itself can cause emphysema because of a decrease in the lungs' elastic recoil ability.

Thoracic cavity

The thoracic cavity is an area that's surrounded by the diaphragm (below), the scalene muscles and fasciae of the neck (above), and the ribs, intercostal muscles, vertebrae, sternum, and ligaments (around the circumference).

Thoracic cage

Anterior thoracic cage

The anterior thoracic cage consists of the manubrium, sternum, xiphoid process, and ribs. It protects the mediastinal organs that lie between the right and left pleural cavities.

Above the anterior thorax is a depression called the **suprasternal notch.** Because the suprasternal notch isn't covered by the rib cage like the rest of the thorax, the trachea and aortic pulsation can be palpated here.

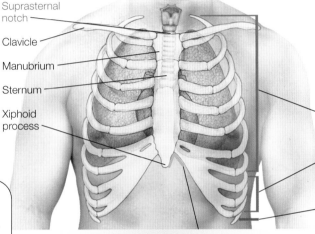

Suprasternal notch

Clavicle

Manubrium

Sternum

Xiphoid process

Ribs 1 through 7 attach directly to the sternum.

Ribs 8 through 10 attach to the cartilage of the preceding rib.

The other two pairs of ribs are "free-floating"—they don't attach to any part of the anterior thoracic cage. Rib 11 ends anterolaterally, as shown here. Rib 12 ends laterally (not visible in this image).

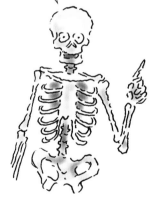

Composed of bone and cartilage, the thoracic cage supports and protects the lungs, allowing them to expand and contract.

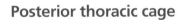

The lower parts of the rib cage (costal margins) near the xiphoid process form the borders of the **costal angle**— an angle of about 90 degrees in a normal person.

Posterior thoracic cage

The vertebral column and 12 pairs of ribs form the posterior portion of the thoracic cage.

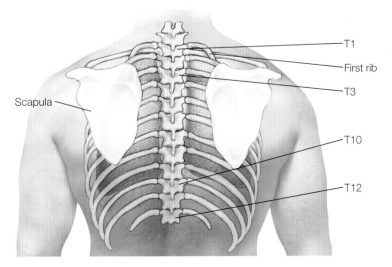

T1

First rib

T3

Scapula

T10

T12

Inspiration and expiration

Breathing involves two actions: inspiration (an active process) and expiration (a relatively passive process). Both actions rely on respiratory muscle function and the effects of pressure differences in the lungs.

Inspiration

During inspiration, the diaphragm contracts (pressing the abdominal organs downward and forward) and the external intercostal muscles also contract. The rib cage expands, the volume of the thoracic cavity increases, and air rushes in to equalize the pressure.

Left lung

External intercostal muscles

Expiration

During expiration, the lungs passively recoil as the diaphragm and intercostal muscles relax, pushing air out of the lungs.

Left lung

Internal intercostal muscles

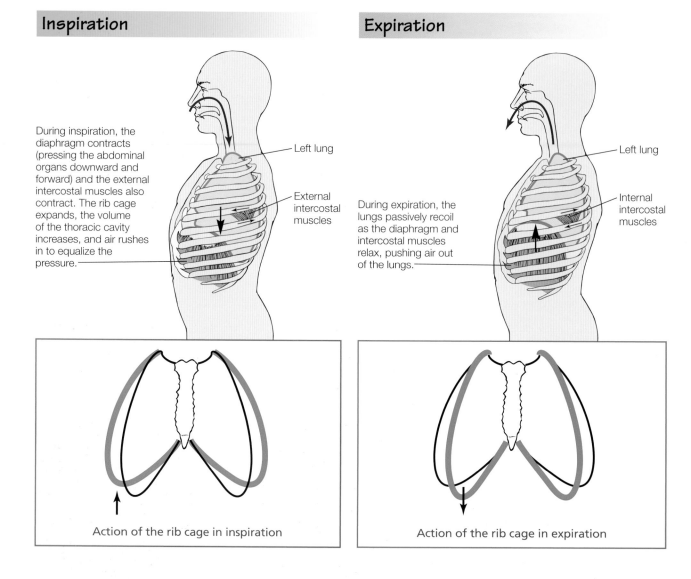

Action of the rib cage in inspiration

Action of the rib cage in expiration

External and internal respiration

Effective respiration requires gas exchange in the lungs (*external respiration*) and gas exchange in the tissues (*internal respiration*).

External respiration occurs through three processes:

 ventilation—gas distribution into and out of the pulmonary airways

pulmonary perfusion—blood flow from the right side of the heart, through the pulmonary circulation, and into the left side of the heart

diffusion—gas movement through a semipermeable membrane from an area of greater concentration to one of lesser concentration.

Ventilation

Ventilation is the distribution of gases (oxygen and carbon dioxide) into and out of the pulmonary airways. Airflow distribution can be affected by:

- airflow pattern
- volume and location of the functional reserve capacity (air retained in the alveoli that prevents their collapse during respiration)
- degree of intrapulmonary resistance
- presence of lung disease.

If airflow is disrupted, airflow distribution follows the path of least resistance.

Comparing airflow patterns

The pattern of airflow through the respiratory passages affects airway resistance.

Laminar flow

Laminar flow, a linear pattern that occurs at low flow rates, offers minimal resistance. This flow type occurs mainly in the small peripheral airways of the bronchial tree.

Turbulent flow

The eddying pattern of turbulent flow creates friction and increases resistance. Turbulent flow is normal in the trachea and large central bronchi. If the smaller airways become constricted or clogged with secretions, however, turbulent flow may also occur there.

Transitional flow

A mixed pattern known as transitional flow is common at lower flow rates in the larger airways, especially where the airways narrow from obstruction, meet, or branch.

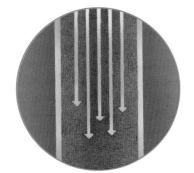

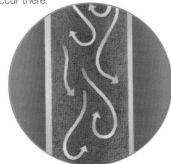

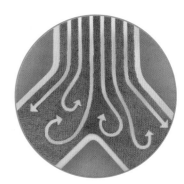

Pulmonary perfusion

In pulmonary perfusion, the right ventricle powers blood flow from the right side of the heart through the lungs and into the left side of the heart.

1 The right and left pulmonary arteries carry deoxygenated blood from the right ventricle to the lungs.

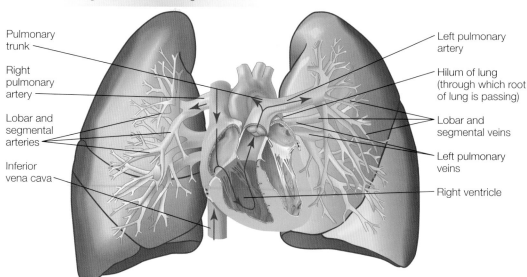

2 These arteries divide to form distal branches called *arterioles*, which terminate as a concentrated capillary network in the alveoli and alveolar sac, where gas exchange occurs.

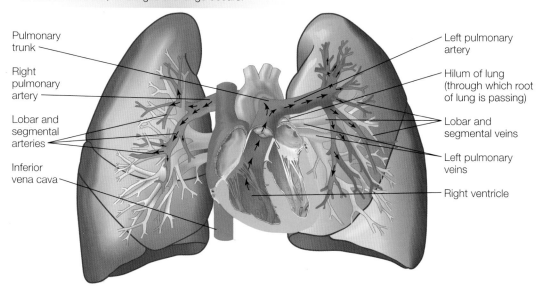

3 Venules—the end branches of the pulmonary veins—collect oxygenated blood from the capillaries and transport it to larger vessels, which carry it to the pulmonary veins.

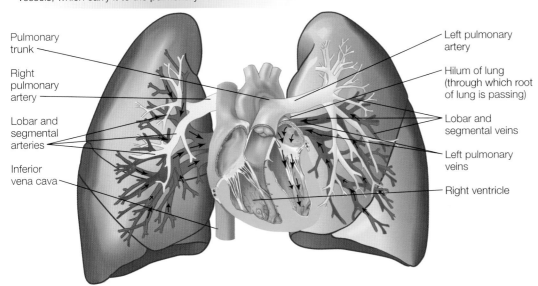

Pulmonary trunk

Right pulmonary artery

Lobar and segmental arteries

Inferior vena cava

Left pulmonary artery

Hilum of lung (through which root of lung is passing)

Lobar and segmental veins

Left pulmonary veins

Right ventricle

4 The pulmonary veins enter the left side of the heart, and the left ventricle distributes oxygenated blood throughout the body.

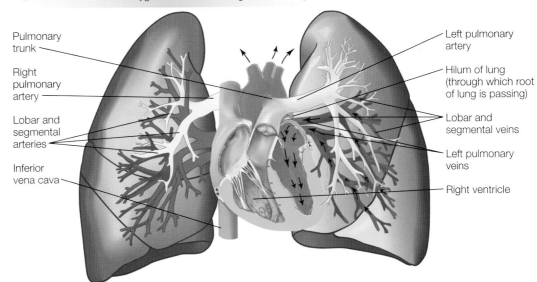

Pulmonary trunk

Right pulmonary artery

Lobar and segmental arteries

Inferior vena cava

Left pulmonary artery

Hilum of lung (through which root of lung is passing)

Lobar and segmental veins

Left pulmonary veins

Right ventricle

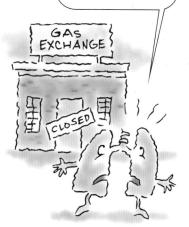

When we all work together, gas exchange goes off without a hitch!

RETURNS & EXCHANGES

Diffusion

Blood in the pulmonary capillaries gains oxygen and loses carbon dioxide through the process of diffusion. In this process, oxygen and carbon dioxide move from an area of greater concentration to an area of lesser concentration through the pulmonary capillary. This illustration shows how the differences in gas concentration between blood in the pulmonary artery (deoxygenated blood from the right side of the heart) and alveolus make this process possible. Gas concentrations depicted in the pulmonary vein are the end result of gas exchange and represent the blood that's delivered to the left side of the heart and systemic circulation.

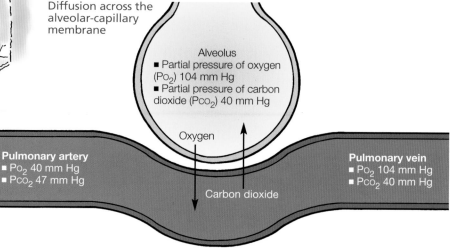

Diffusion across the alveolar-capillary membrane

Alveolus
- Partial pressure of oxygen (P_{O_2}) 104 mm Hg
- Partial pressure of carbon dioxide (P_{CO_2}) 40 mm Hg

Oxygen

Carbon dioxide

Pulmonary artery
- P_{O_2} 40 mm Hg
- P_{CO_2} 47 mm Hg

Pulmonary vein
- P_{O_2} 104 mm Hg
- P_{CO_2} 40 mm Hg

Pulmonary capillary

When gas exchange doesn't work, we're all in for hard times!

GAS EXCHANGE

CLOSED

Ventilation-perfusion ratio

Gravity can affect oxygen and carbon dioxide transport in a positive way. It causes unoxygenated blood to travel more to the lower and middle lung lobes than to the upper lobes. This explains why ventilation and perfusion differ in the various parts of the lungs.

Areas where perfusion and ventilation are similar have a ventilation-perfusion ($\dot{V}/\dot{Q}$) match. Gas exchange is most efficient in such areas. For example, in normal lung function, the alveoli receive air at a rate of about 4 L/minute, while the capillaries supply blood to the alveoli at a rate of about 5 L/minute, creating a $\dot{V}/\dot{Q}$ ratio of 4:5, or 0.8 (normal $\dot{V}/\dot{Q}$ ratio range is 0.8 to 1.2).

A $\dot{V}/\dot{Q}$ mismatch indicates ineffective gas exchange between the alveoli and pulmonary capillaries. Such a mismatch can affect all body systems by changing the amount of oxygen delivered to living cells.

What happens in ventilation-perfusion mismatch

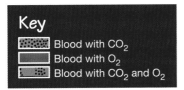

Key
- Blood with CO_2
- Blood with O_2
- Blood with CO_2 and O_2

Causes

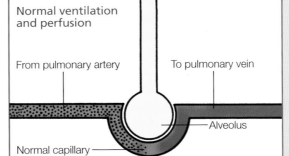

Normal ventilation and perfusion

From pulmonary artery

To pulmonary vein

Alveolus

Normal capillary

With a $\dot{V}/\dot{Q}$ match, unoxygenated blood from the venous system returns to the right side of the heart through the pulmonary artery to the lungs, carrying carbon dioxide. The arteries branch into the alveolar capillaries, where gas exchange takes place.

1 **Shunting** (reduced ventilation to a lung unit) causes unoxygenated blood to move from the right side of the heart to the left side of the heart and into systemic circulation; it may result from physical defects or airway obstruction.

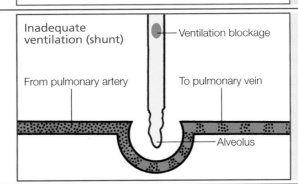

Inadequate ventilation (shunt)

Ventilation blockage

From pulmonary artery

To pulmonary vein

Alveolus

When the $\dot{V}/\dot{Q}$ ratio is low, pulmonary circulation is adequate but not enough oxygen is available to the alveoli for normal diffusion. A portion of the blood flowing through the pulmonary vessels doesn't become oxygenated.

2 **Dead-space ventilation** (reduced perfusion to a lung unit) occurs when alveoli don't have adequate blood supply for gas exchange to occur, such as with pulmonary emboli and pulmonary infarction.

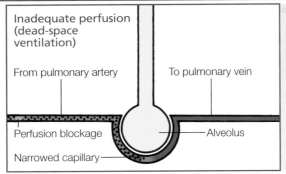

Inadequate perfusion (dead-space ventilation)

From pulmonary artery

To pulmonary vein

Perfusion blockage

Alveolus

Narrowed capillary

When the $\dot{V}/\dot{Q}$ ratio is high, ventilation is normal but alveolar perfusion is reduced or absent. Note the narrowed capillary, indicating poor perfusion. This commonly results from a perfusion defect, such as pulmonary embolism or a disorder that decreases cardiac output.

3 A **silent unit** (a combination of shunting and dead-space ventilation) occurs when little or no ventilation and perfusion are present, such as in cases of pneumothorax and acute respiratory distress syndrome.

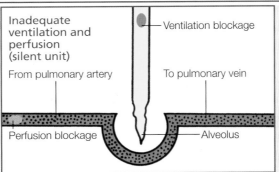

Inadequate ventilation and perfusion (silent unit)

Ventilation blockage

From pulmonary artery

To pulmonary vein

Perfusion blockage

Alveolus

The silent unit indicates an absence of ventilation and perfusion to the lung area. The silent unit may help compensate for a $\dot{V}/\dot{Q}$ imbalance by delivering blood flow to better ventilated lung areas.

VISION QUEST

Able to label?

Identify the paranasal sinuses in this illustration.

1._____
2._____
3._____

Show and tell

Describe the mechanics of breathing using the illustrations here as a guide.

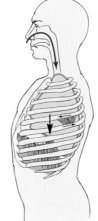

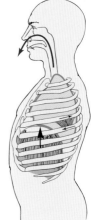

1._____
_____
_____
_____
_____

2._____
_____
_____
_____
_____

Answers: Able to label? 1. Frontal, 2. Ethmoidal, 3. Maxillary. Show and tell 1. During inspiration, the diaphragm contracts (pressing the abdominal organs downward and forward), and the external intercostal muscles also contract. The rib cage expands, the volume of the thoracic cavity increases, and air rushes in to equalize the pressure. 2. During expiration, the lungs passively recoil as the diaphragm and intercostal muscles relax, pushing air out of the lungs.

13 Gastrointestinal system

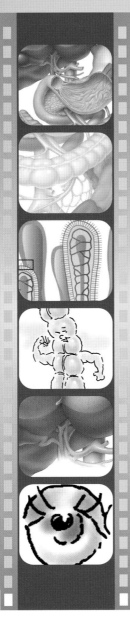

- GI system basics 152
- Alimentary canal 152
- GI tract innervation 159
- Accessory organs of digestion 160
- Digestion and elimination 164
- Vision quest 170

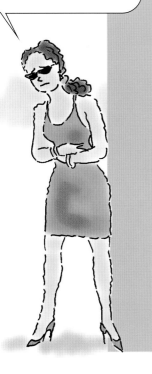

I've always thought performing gave me butterflies in my stomach. But, after reading this chapter, I'm wondering whether it isn't my digestion.

GI system basics

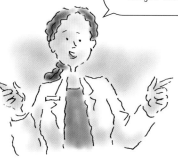

The GI system has two major components and two major functions.

GI components

- Alimentary canal (also called the *GI tract*)
- Accessory GI organs

GI functions

- Digestion (breaking down food and fluid into simple chemicals that can be absorbed into the bloodstream and transported throughout the body)
- Elimination of waste products (through excretion of stool)

Alimentary canal

The alimentary canal is a hollow muscular tube that begins in the mouth and extends to the anus.

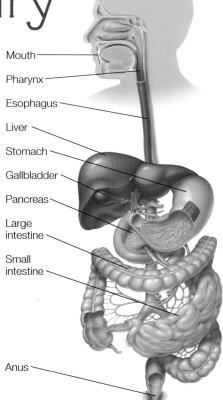

- Mouth
- Pharynx
- Esophagus
- Liver
- Stomach
- Gallbladder
- Pancreas
- Large intestine
- Small intestine
- Anus

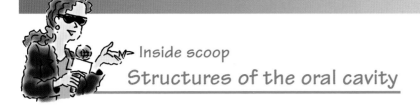

Inside scoop

Structures of the oral cavity

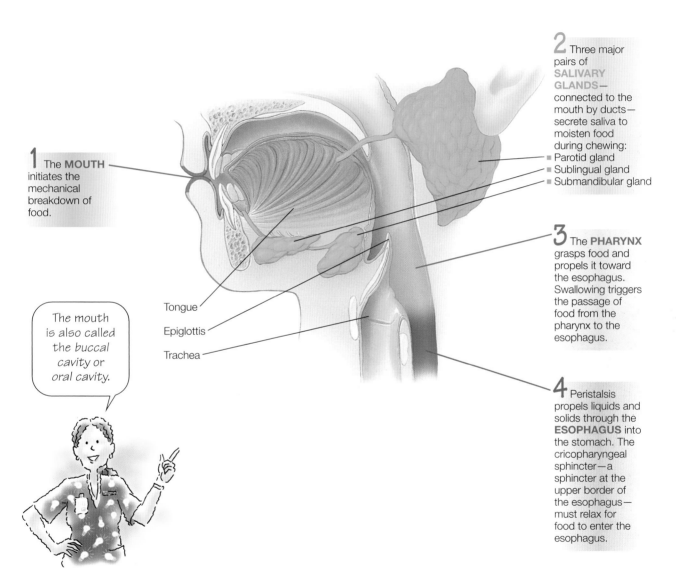

1 The **MOUTH** initiates the mechanical breakdown of food.

The mouth is also called the buccal cavity or oral cavity.

Tongue

Epiglottis

Trachea

2 Three major pairs of **SALIVARY GLANDS**— connected to the mouth by ducts— secrete saliva to moisten food during chewing:
- Parotid gland
- Sublingual gland
- Submandibular gland

3 The **PHARYNX** grasps food and propels it toward the esophagus. Swallowing triggers the passage of food from the pharynx to the esophagus.

4 Peristalsis propels liquids and solids through the **ESOPHAGUS** into the stomach. The cricopharyngeal sphincter—a sphincter at the upper border of the esophagus— must relax for food to enter the esophagus.

Stomach

The stomach is a collapsible, saclike structure.

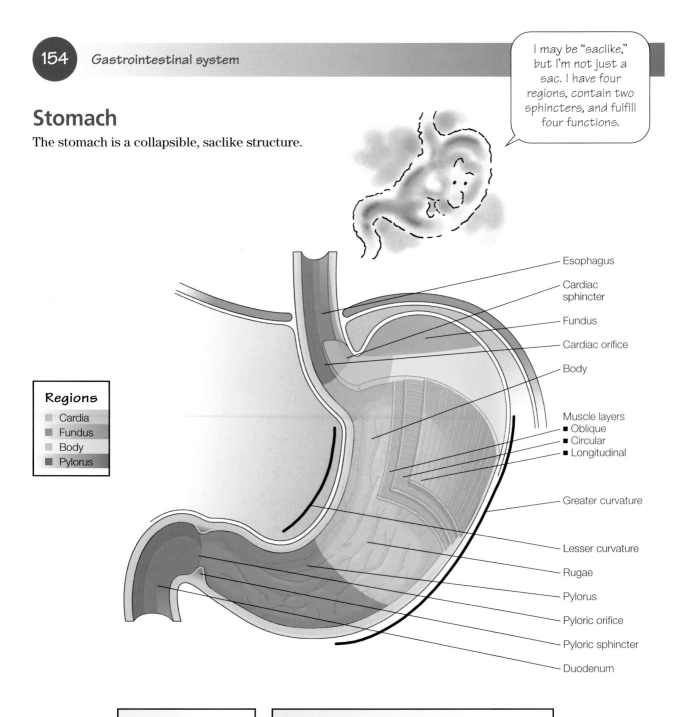

I may be "saclike," but I'm not just a sac. I have four regions, contain two sphincters, and fulfill four functions.

Esophagus

Cardiac sphincter

Fundus

Cardiac orifice

Body

Muscle layers
- Oblique
- Circular
- Longitudinal

Greater curvature

Lesser curvature

Rugae

Pylorus

Pyloric orifice

Pyloric sphincter

Duodenum

Regions

- Cardia
- Fundus
- Body
- Pylorus

Sphincters

- Cardiac (protects the entrance to the stomach)
- Pyloric (guards the exit to the duodenum)

Functions

- Serves as a temporary storage area for food
- Begins digestion
- Breaks down food into chyme, a semifluid substance
- Moves gastric contents into the small intestine

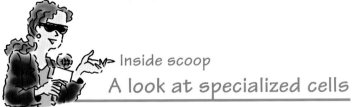

Inside scoop

A look at specialized cells

Specialized cells throughout the GI tract
aid digestion and excretion.

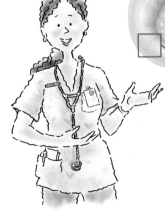

Digestion is truly a
process. Food entering the
stomach triggers the release
of gastrin, a hormone that
aids digestion. Then, as
chyme moves from the
stomach to the duodenum,
secretin is released.

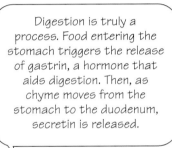

Stomach

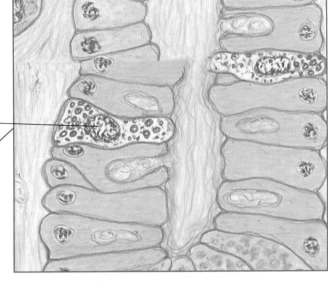

G cells in
pyloric
glands
(secrete
gastrin)

Duodenum and jejunum

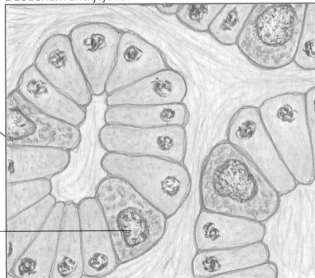

S cells in
duodenal
and
jejunal
glands
(secrete
secretin)

Small intestine

The small intestine is a tube that measures about 20′ (6 m) long. It's the longest organ of the GI tract.

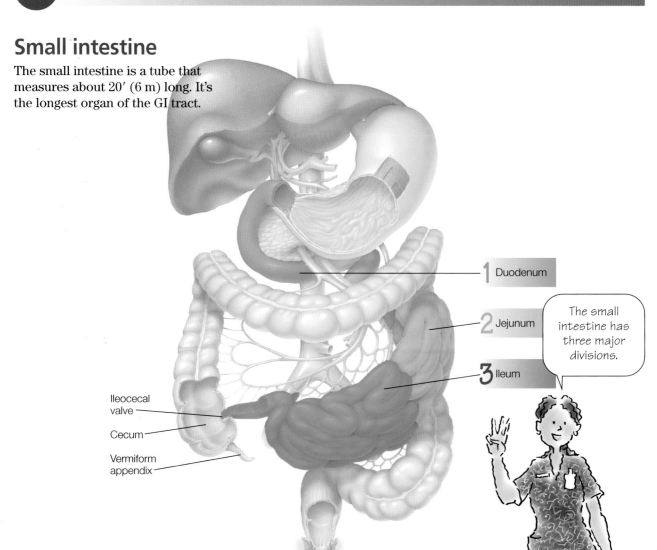

1 Duodenum

2 Jejunum

3 Ileum

The small intestine has three major divisions.

Ileocecal valve

Cecum

Vermiform appendix

Functions

■ Completes food digestion
■ Absorbs food molecules through its wall into the circulatory system, which then delivers them to body cells
■ Secretes hormones that help control secretion of bile, pancreatic juice, and intestinal juice

More than meets the eye

The intestinal wall has structural features that significantly increase its absorptive surface area. These include:
■ villi—fingerlike projections on the mucosa
■ microvilli—tiny cytoplasmic projections on the surface of epithelial cells.

Other structures found in the small intestines include:
■ intestinal crypts—simple glands lodged in the grooves separating villi
■ Peyer's patches—collections of lymphatic tissue within the submucosa
■ Brunner's glands—glands that secrete mucus.

Large intestine

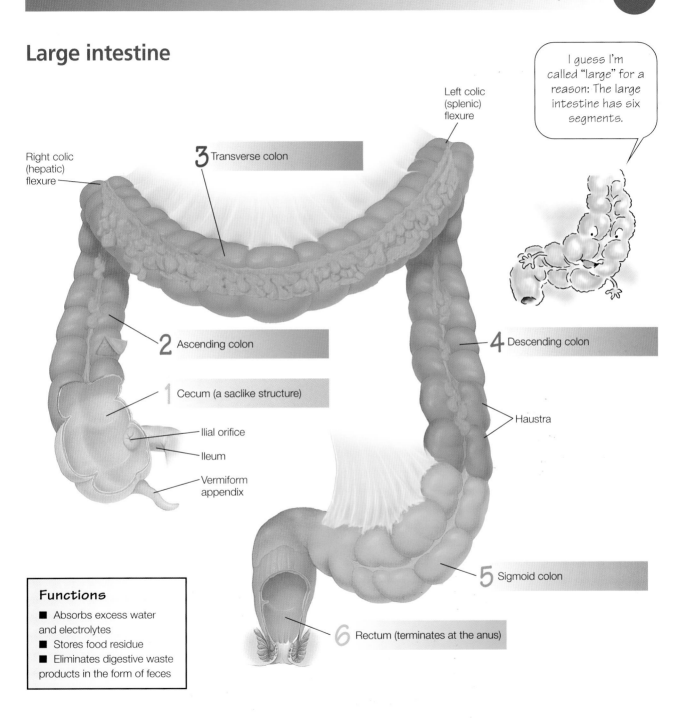

I guess I'm called "large" for a reason: The large intestine has six segments.

Left colic (splenic) flexure

Right colic (hepatic) flexure

3 Transverse colon

2 Ascending colon

4 Descending colon

1 Cecum (a saclike structure)

Ilial orifice

Ileum

Vermiform appendix

Haustra

5 Sigmoid colon

6 Rectum (terminates at the anus)

Functions
- Absorbs excess water and electrolytes
- Stores food residue
- Eliminates digestive waste products in the form of feces

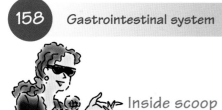

→ Inside scoop

Let's look at the layers of the GI tract, starting with the visceral peritoneum (the outermost layer) all the way down to the mucosa (the innermost layer).

GI tract wall structures

Tunica muscularis
- Composed of skeletal muscle in the mouth, pharynx, and upper esophagus
- Circular fibers thicken to form sphincters
- Taeniae coli pucker the large intestine into characteristic pouches (haustra)

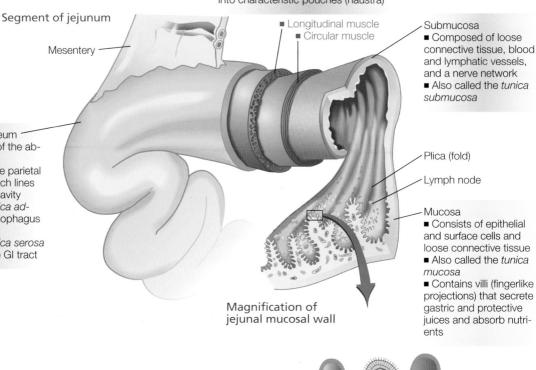

Segment of jejunum

Mesentery

- Longitudinal muscle
- Circular muscle

Submucosa
- Composed of loose connective tissue, blood and lymphatic vessels, and a nerve network
- Also called the *tunica submucosa*

Visceral peritoneum
- Covers most of the abdominal organs
- Lies next to the parietal peritoneum, which lines the abdominal cavity
- Called the *tunica adventitia* in the esophagus and rectum
- Called the *tunica serosa* elsewhere in the GI tract

Plica (fold)

Lymph node

Mucosa
- Consists of epithelial and surface cells and loose connective tissue
- Also called the *tunica mucosa*
- Contains villi (fingerlike projections) that secrete gastric and protective juices and absorb nutrients

Magnification of jejunal mucosal wall

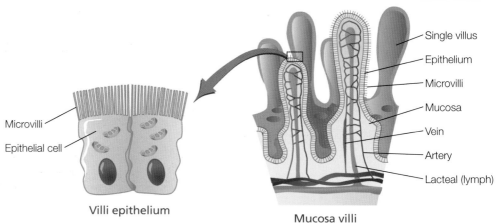

Microvilli

Epithelial cell

Villi epithelium

Single villus

Epithelium

Microvilli

Mucosa

Vein

Artery

Lacteal (lymph)

Mucosa villi

GI tract innervation

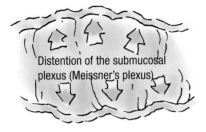

Distention of the submucosal plexus (Meissner's plexus)

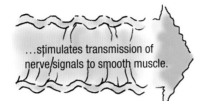

…stimulates transmission of nerve signals to smooth muscle.

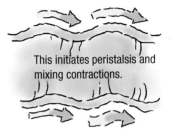

This initiates peristalsis and mixing contractions.

Parasympathetic stimulation

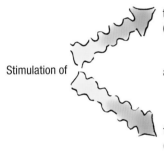

Stimulation of

the vagus nerve (for most of the intestines)

and

the sacral spinal nerves (for the descending colon and rectum)

increases gut and sphincter tone.

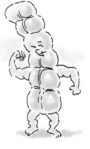

This increases the frequency, strength, and velocity of smooth-muscle contractions as well as motor secretory activities.

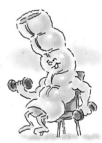

Sympathetic stimulation

Stimulation of

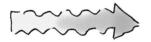

spinal nerves

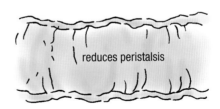

reduces peristalsis

and reduces GI activity.

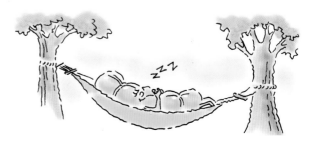

Accessory organs of digestion

Accessory organs include the liver, biliary duct system, and pancreas. These organs contribute hormones, enzymes, and bile, which are vital to digestion.

Liver

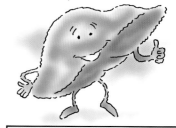

Not to brag, but I am the largest gland in the body.

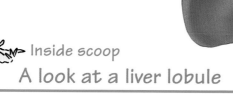

Inside scoop
A look at a liver lobule

The liver's functional unit is called a *lobule.* It consists of a plate of hepatic cells, or *hepatocytes,* that encircle a central vein and radiate outward. Separating the hepatocyte plates from each other are *sinusoids,* which serve as the liver's capillary system. Sinusoids carry oxygenated blood from the hepatic artery and nutrient-rich blood from the portal vein.

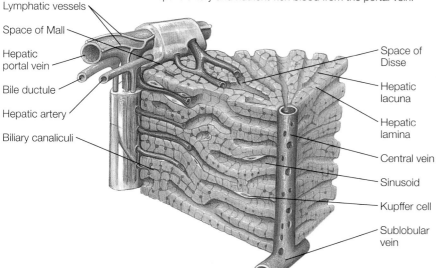

Lymphatic vessels
Space of Mall
Hepatic portal vein
Bile ductule
Hepatic artery
Biliary canaliculi

Space of Disse
Hepatic lacuna
Hepatic lamina
Central vein
Sinusoid
Kupffer cell
Sublobular vein

Functions
- Metabolizes carbohydrates, fats, and proteins
- Detoxifies blood
- Converts ammonia to urea for excretion
- Synthesizes plasma proteins, nonessential amino acids, vitamins, and essential nutrients
- Secretes bile

Biliary duct system

Think of the ducts as a subway system transporting bile through the GI tract.

Functions of bile

■ Emulsifies fat
■ Promotes intestinal absorption of fatty acids, cholesterol, and other lipids
■ Gives stool its color

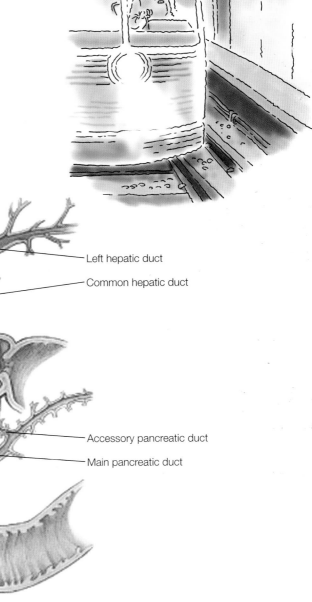

Right hepatic duct

Gallbladder

Cystic duct

Common bile duct

Minor duodenal papilla

Sphincter of ampulla

Major duodenal papilla

Left hepatic duct

Common hepatic duct

Accessory pancreatic duct

Main pancreatic duct

GI hormones: Production and function

When stimulated, GI structures secrete five hormones. Each hormone plays a different role in digestion.

Hormone and production site	Stimulating factor or agent	Function
Gastrin Produced in pyloric antrum and duodenal mucosa	▪ Pyloric antrum distention ▪ Vagal stimulation ▪ Protein digestion products ▪ Alcohol	Stimulates gastric secretion and motility
Gastric inhibitory peptides Produced in duodenal and jejunal mucosa	▪ Gastric acid ▪ Fats ▪ Fat digestion products	Inhibits gastric secretion and motility
Secretin Produced in duodenal and jejunal mucosa	▪ Gastric acid ▪ Fat digestion products ▪ Protein digestion products	Stimulates secretion of bile and alkaline pancreatic fluid
Cholecystokinin Produced in duodenal and jejunal mucosa	▪ Fat digestion products ▪ Protein digestion products	Stimulates gallbladder contraction and secretion of enzyme-rich pancreatic fluid
Motilin Produced in duodenal mucosa	▪ Gastric acid ▪ Fats	Increases gastric motility

Gallbladder and pancreas

Together the gallbladder and pancreas constitute the biliary tract.

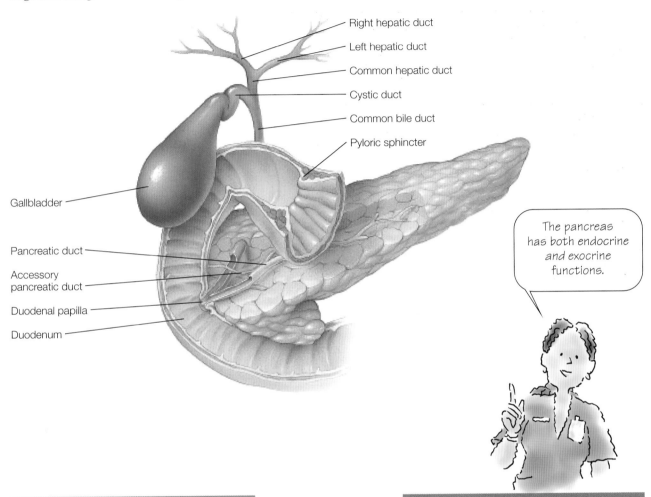

Right hepatic duct
Left hepatic duct
Common hepatic duct
Cystic duct
Common bile duct
Pyloric sphincter
Gallbladder
Pancreatic duct
Accessory pancreatic duct
Duodenal papilla
Duodenum

The pancreas has both endocrine and exocrine functions.

Gallbladder

- Pear-shaped organ joined to the ventral surface of the liver by the cystic duct
- Covered with visceral peritoneum
- Stores and concentrates bile produced by the liver
- Releases bile into the common bile duct for delivery to the duodenum in response to the contraction and relaxation of Oddi's sphincter

Pancreas

- Measures 6″ to 8″ (15 to 20.5 cm) in length
- Consists of a head, body, and tail
- Beta cells secrete insulin to promote carbohydrate metabolism (endocrine function)
- Alpha cells secrete glucagon to stimulate glycogenolysis in the liver (endocrine function)
- Produces enzymes that aid in digestion (exocrine function)

Digestion and elimination

1. Digestion starts in the oral cavity, where chewing *(mastication)*, salivation (the beginning of starch digestion), and swallowing *(deglutition)* all take place.

2. When a person swallows, the hypopharyngeal sphincter in the upper esophagus relaxes, allowing food to enter the esophagus.

3. After the food is in the esophagus, the glossopharyngeal nerve activates peristalsis, which moves the food down toward the stomach.

4. As food passes through the esophagus, glands in the esophageal mucosal layer secrete mucus, which lubricates the bolus and protects the mucosal membrane from damage caused by poorly chewed foods.

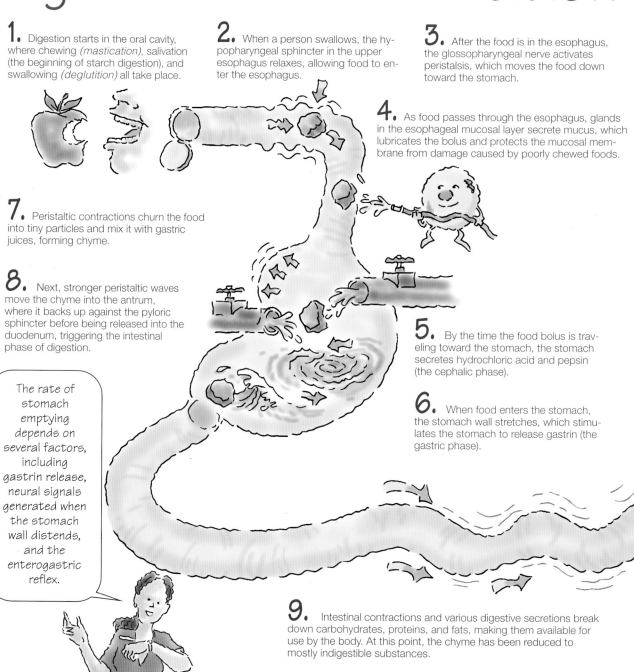

7. Peristaltic contractions churn the food into tiny particles and mix it with gastric juices, forming chyme.

8. Next, stronger peristaltic waves move the chyme into the antrum, where it backs up against the pyloric sphincter before being released into the duodenum, triggering the intestinal phase of digestion.

The rate of stomach emptying depends on several factors, including gastrin release, neural signals generated when the stomach wall distends, and the enterogastric reflex.

5. By the time the food bolus is traveling toward the stomach, the stomach secretes hydrochloric acid and pepsin (the cephalic phase).

6. When food enters the stomach, the stomach wall stretches, which stimulates the stomach to release gastrin (the gastric phase).

9. Intestinal contractions and various digestive secretions break down carbohydrates, proteins, and fats, making them available for use by the body. At this point, the chyme has been reduced to mostly indigestible substances.

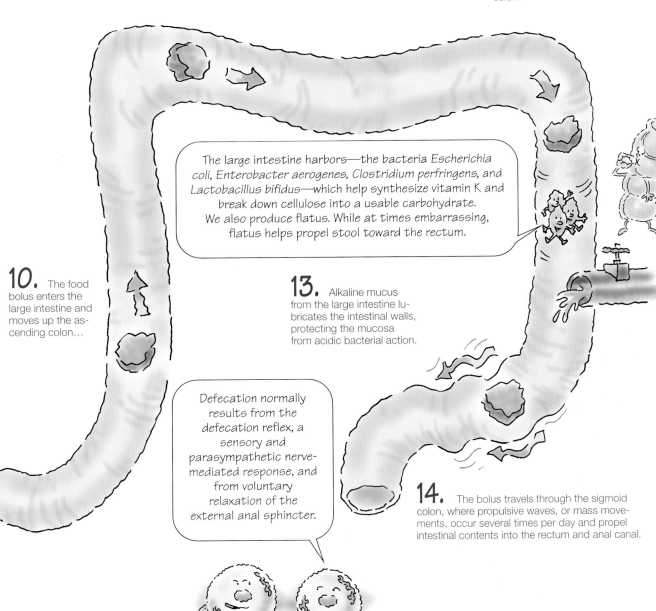

11. …across the transverse colon…

12. …and down through the descending colon.

The large intestine harbors—the bacteria *Escherichia coli, Enterobacter aerogenes, Clostridium perfringens,* and *Lactobacillus bifidus*—which help synthesize vitamin K and break down cellulose into a usable carbohydrate. We also produce flatus. While at times embarrassing, flatus helps propel stool toward the rectum.

10. The food bolus enters the large intestine and moves up the ascending colon…

13. Alkaline mucus from the large intestine lubricates the intestinal walls, protecting the mucosa from acidic bacterial action.

Defecation normally results from the defecation reflex, a sensory and parasympathetic nerve-mediated response, and from voluntary relaxation of the external anal sphincter.

14. The bolus travels through the sigmoid colon, where propulsive waves, or mass movements, occur several times per day and propel intestinal contents into the rectum and anal canal.

What happens in swallowing

Before peristalsis can begin, the neural pattern that initiates swallowing must occur. This process is described here and illustrated below:

■ Food pushed to the back of the mouth stimulates swallowing receptor areas that surround the pharyngeal opening.

■ These receptor areas transmit impulses to the brain by way of the sensory portions of the trigeminal and glossopharyngeal nerves.

■ The brain's swallowing center (located in the brainstem) then relays motor impulses to the esophagus by way of the trigeminal, glossopharyngeal, vagus, and hypoglossal nerves, causing swallowing to occur.

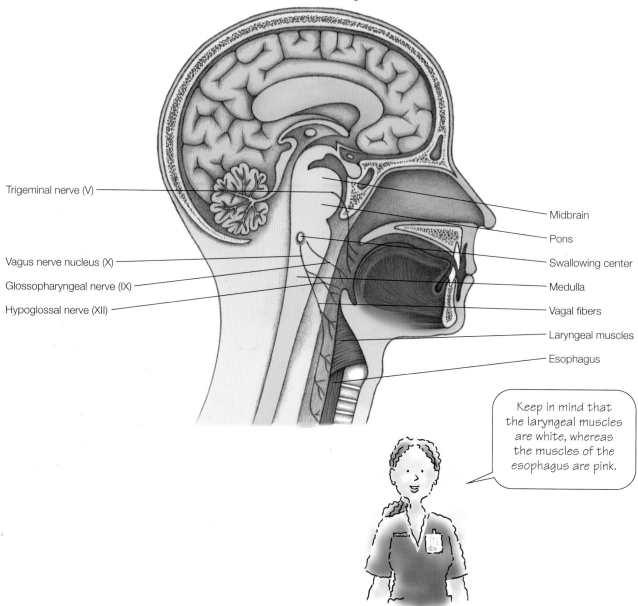

Trigeminal nerve (V)

Vagus nerve nucleus (X)

Glossopharyngeal nerve (IX)

Hypoglossal nerve (XII)

Midbrain

Pons

Swallowing center

Medulla

Vagal fibers

Laryngeal muscles

Esophagus

Keep in mind that the laryngeal muscles are white, whereas the muscles of the esophagus are pink.

Sites and mechanisms of gastric secretion

The body of the stomach lies between the lower esophageal sphincter (LES), or cardiac sphincter, and the pyloric sphincter. Between these sphincters lie the fundus, body, antrum, and pylorus. These areas have a rich variety of mucosal cells that help the stomach carry out its tasks.

Glands and gastric secretions

Cardiac glands, pyloric glands, and gastric glands secrete 2 to 3 L of gastric juice daily through the stomach's gastric pits. Here are the details:

■ Both the cardiac gland (near the LES) and the pyloric gland (near the pylorus) secrete thin mucus.

■ The gastric gland (in the body and fundus) secretes hydrochloric acid (HCl), pepsinogen, intrinsic factor, and mucus.

Protection from self-digestion

Specialized cells line the gastric glands, gastric pits, and surface epithelium. Mucous cells in the necks of the gastric glands produce thin mucus. Mucous cells in the surface epithelium produce an alkaline mucus. Both substances lubricate food and protect the stomach from self-digestion by corrosive enzymes.

Other secretions

Argentaffin cells produce gastrin, which stimulates gastric secretion and motility. Chief cells produce pepsinogen, which breaks proteins down into polypeptides. Large parietal cells scattered throughout the fundus secrete HCl and intrinsic factor. HCl degrades pepsinogen, maintains acid environment, and inhibits excess bacteria growth. Intrinsic factor promotes vitamin B_{12} absorption in the small intestine.

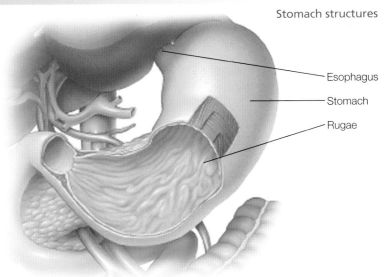

Stomach structures

— Esophagus

— Stomach

— Rugae

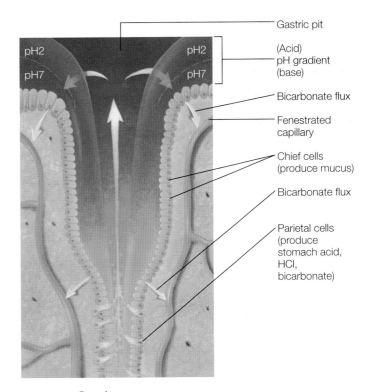

Gastric pit

(Acid)
pH gradient
(base)

Bicarbonate flux

Fenestrated capillary

Chief cells (produce mucus)

Bicarbonate flux

Parietal cells (produce stomach acid, HCl, bicarbonate)

pH2   pH2
pH7   pH7

Gastric mucosa

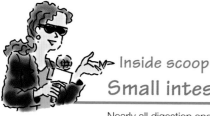

Inside scoop

Small intestine: How form affects absorption

Nearly all digestion and absorption take place in the 20' (6.1 m) of small intestine. The structure of the small intestine is key to digestion and absorption.

Specialized mucosa

Multiple projections of the intestinal mucosa increase the surface area for absorption several hundredfold, as shown in the enlarged views at right.

Circular projections (*Kerckring's folds*) are covered by villi. Each villus contains a lymphatic vessel (*lacteal*), a venule, capillaries, an arteriole, nerve fibers, and smooth muscle.

Each villus is densely fringed with about 2,000 microvilli, making it resemble a fine brush. The villi are lined with columnar epithelial cells, which dip into the lamina propria between the villi to form intestinal glands (*crypts of Lieberkühn*).

Types of epithelial cells

The type of epithelial cell dictates its function. Mucus-secreting goblet cells are found on and between the villi on the crypt mucosa. In the proximal duodenum, specialized Brunner's glands also secrete large amounts of mucus to lubricate and protect the duodenum from potentially corrosive acidic chyme and gastric juices.

Duodenal *argentaffin cells* produce the hormones secretin and cholecystokinin. *Undifferentiated cells* deep within the intestinal glands replace the epithelium. *Absorptive cells* consist of large numbers of tightly packed microvilli over a plasma membrane that contains transport mechanisms for absorption and produces enzymes for the final step in digestion.

Intestinal glands

The intestinal glands primarily secrete a watery fluid that bathes the villi with chyme particles. Fluid production results from local irritation of nerve cells and, possibly, from hormonal stimulation by secretin and cholecystokinin. The microvillous brush border secretes various hormones and digestive enzymes that catalyze final nutrient breakdown.

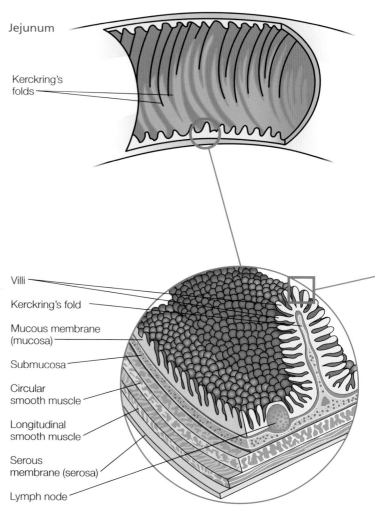

Jejunum

Kerckring's folds

Villi

Kerckring's fold

Mucous membrane (mucosa)

Submucosa

Circular smooth muscle

Longitudinal smooth muscle

Serous membrane (serosa)

Lymph node

Detail of villi

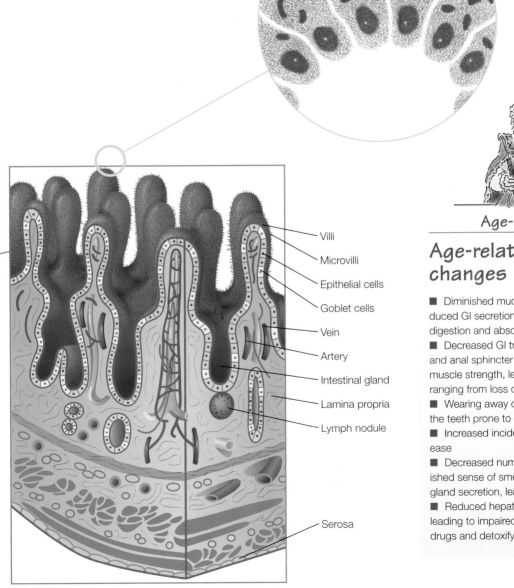

Microvilli brush border

Villi

Microvilli

Epithelial cells

Goblet cells

Vein

Artery

Intestinal gland

Lamina propria

Lymph nodule

Serosa

Detail of intestinal mucosa

Age-old story

Age-related GI changes

■ Diminished mucosal elasticity and reduced GI secretions, leading to impaired digestion and absorption

■ Decreased GI tract motility, bowel wall and anal sphincter tone, and abdominal muscle strength, leading to complaints ranging from loss of appetite to constipation

■ Wearing away of tooth enamel, leaving the teeth prone to cavities

■ Increased incidence of periodontal disease

■ Decreased number of taste buds, diminished sense of smell, and decreased salivary gland secretion, leading to appetite loss

■ Reduced hepatic enzyme production, leading to impaired ability to metabolize drugs and detoxify substances

VISION QUEST

Able to label?

Identify the parts of the small intestine indicated in this illustration.

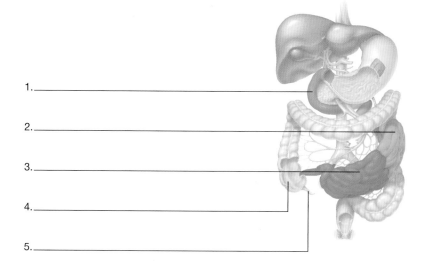

1. _____

2. _____

3. _____

4. _____

5. _____

Matchmaker

Match each of the organs shown with its major function.

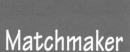

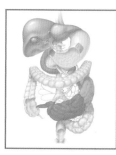

A. Detoxifies blood
B. Completes food digestion
C. Stores and concentrates bile
D. Serves as a temporary storage area for food
E. Absorbs excess water and electrolytes

1. ____

2. ____

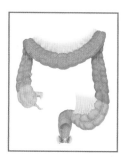

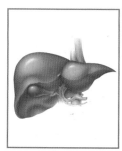

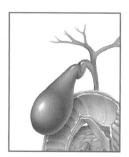

3. ____

4. ____

5. ____

Answers: Able to label? 1. Duodenum, 2. Jejunum, 3. Ileum, 4. Cecum, 5. Vermiform appendix. Matchmaker 1. D, 2. B, 3. E, 4. A, 5. C.

14
Nutrition and metabolism

- Components of nutrition 172
- Digestion and absorption 179
- Metabolism 182
- Vision quest 190

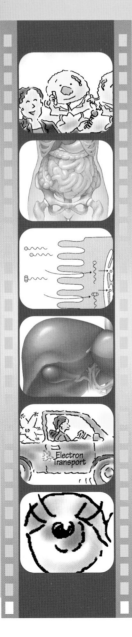

Creative energy requires a combination of inspiration and hard work; physical energy requires a combination of nutrition and metabolism.

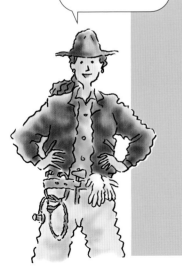

Components of nutrition

Nutrition refers to the intake, assimilation, and utilization of nutrients.

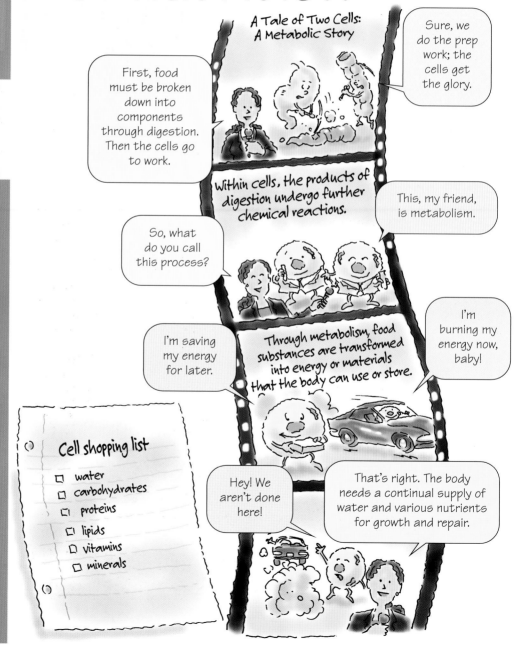

Food group recommendations

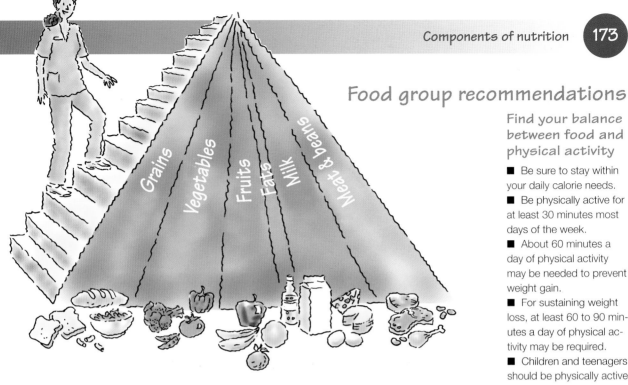

Find your balance between food and physical activity

- Be sure to stay within your daily calorie needs.
- Be physically active for at least 30 minutes most days of the week.
- About 60 minutes a day of physical activity may be needed to prevent weight gain.
- For sustaining weight loss, at least 60 to 90 minutes a day of physical activity may be required.
- Children and teenagers should be physically active for 60 minutes every day, or most days.

Know the limits on fats, sugars, and salt (sodium)

- Make the most of your fat sources from fish, nuts, and vegetable oils.
- Limit solid fats like butter, stick margarine, shortening, and lard, as well as foods that contain these.
- Check the Nutrition Facts label to keep saturated fats, trans fats, and sodium low.
- Choose food and beverages low in added sugars. Added sugars contribute calories with few, if any, nutrients.

Grains	Vegetables	Fruits	Milk	Meats & beans
■ Make one-half of your grains whole. ■ Eat at least 3 oz of whole-grain cereals, breads, crackers, rice, or pasta every day. ■ 1 oz is about 1 slice of bread, about 1 cup of breakfast cereal, or ½ cup of cooked rice, cereal, or pasta.	■ Vary your veggies. ■ Eat more dark-green veggies like broccoli, spinach, and other dark leafy greens. ■ Eat more orange veggies, like carrots and sweet potatoes. ■ Eat more dry beans and peas like pinto beans, kidney beans, and lentils.	■ Focus on fruits. ■ Eat a variety of fruit. ■ Choose fresh, frozen, canned, or dried fruit. ■ Go easy on fruit juices.	■ Consume calcium-rich foods. ■ Go low-fat or fat-free when you choose milk, yogurt, and other milk products. ■ If you don't or can't consume milk, choose lactose-free products or other calcium sources, such as fortified foods and beverages.	■ Go lean with protein. ■ Choose low-fat or lean meats and poultry. ■ Bake it, broil it, or grill it. ■ Vary your protein routine; choose more fish, beans, peas, nuts, and seeds.

For a 2,000 calorie diet, you need the amounts below from each food group. To find the amounts that are right for you, go to MyPyramid.gov.

Eat 6 oz every day.	Eat 2½ cups every day.	Eat 2 cups every day.	Get 3 cups every day; for kids ages 2 to 8, 2 cups.	Eat 5½ oz every day.

Carbohydrates

Carbohydrates are organic compounds composed of carbon, hydrogen, and oxygen and are stored in muscles and the liver. They can be converted quickly when the body needs energy.

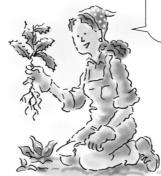

Carbohydrates are made through photosynthesis—the process by which the sun's energy allows chlorophyll-containing plants to take up carbon dioxide through their roots and release oxygen into the air. Carbon and water that remain in the plant form carbohydrates.

Monosaccharides

- Are simple sugars
- Can't be broken down by the digestive process
- Are absorbed through the small intestine
- Examples: glucose (dextrose), fructose, galactose

Disaccharides

- Are synthesized from monosaccharides
- Consist of two monosaccharides minus a water molecule
- Examples: sucrose, lactose, maltose

Polysaccharides

- Are synthesized from monosaccharides
- Are ingested and broken down into simple sugars and used for fuel
- Consist of a long chain of monosaccharides linked by glycoside bonds
- Examples: glycogen, starch

Proteins

Components of every living cell, proteins are large, complex molecules composed of individual building blocks known as *amino acids*.

Protein is:

- required for normal growth and development
- broken down by the body as a source of energy when the supply of carbohydrates and fats is inadequate
- stored in muscle, bone, skin, cartilage, and lymph.

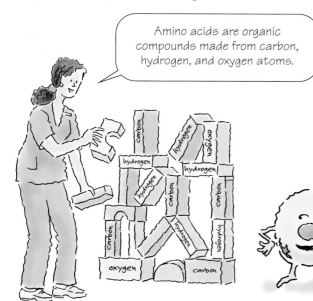

Amino acids are organic compounds made from carbon, hydrogen, and oxygen atoms.

Considering that the shape of a protein molecule determines how it functions, what's this going to be?

Fats

Also known as *lipids*, fats are organic compounds that don't dissolve in water but do dissolve in alcohol and other organic solvents.

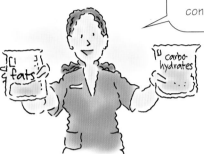

Because fats have less oxygen, they provide more than double the amount of calories than the same amount of carbohydrates. That makes fat a concentrated form of fuel.

Triglycerides

■ Account for about 95% of the fat in food
■ Are the major storage form of fat in the body
■ Contain fatty acids that can be saturated or unsaturated.

Saturated fatty acid

■ Saturated or filled with hydrogen ions
■ Found in meat, poultry, full-fat dairy products, and tropical oils (such as palm and coconut oils).

Unsaturated fatty acid

■ Not completely filled with hydrogen ions
■ Usually soft or liquid at room temperature
■ Originate from plant fat and oils
■ Have lower melting points
■ Can become rancid when exposed to extended periods of light and oxygen

Trans fats

■ Produced by hydrogenation
■ Found in vegetable shortening, certain margarines, crackers, cookies, snack foods, and other foods made with hydrogenated oils

Phospholipids

■ Complex lipids that are similar to fat but that have a phosphorus- and nitrogen-containing compound that replaces one of the fatty acid molecules
■ Are major structural components of cell membranes
■ Occur naturally in all foods

Sterols

■ Complex molecules in which the carbon atoms form four cyclic structures attached to various side chains
■ Contain no glycerol or fatty acid molecules
■ Example: cholesterol

Cholesterol

■ Most common sterol
■ Manufactured daily by the body
■ Produced and filtered by the liver
■ Necessary for the production of some hormones (estrogen, cortisone, adrenaline, and testosterone)

Vitamins and minerals

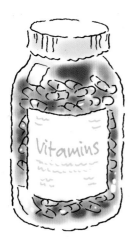

- Organic compounds needed in small quantities for normal metabolism, growth, and development
- Classified as water-soluble or fat-soluble
- Water-soluble vitamins: include B complex and C vitamins
- Fat-soluble vitamins: include vitamins A, D, E, and K

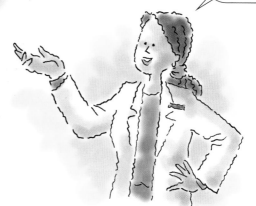

memory board

To remember the fat-soluble vitamins (A, D, E, K), think:

All
Dieters
Enjoy
Kale.

It may not be true, but it will help you remember!

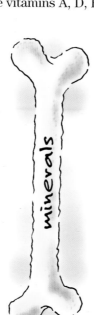

- Inorganic substances found in bones, hemoglobin, thyroxine, and vitamin B
- Play important roles in:
  - enzyme metabolism
  - membrane transfer of essential compounds
  - regulation of acid-base balance
  - osmotic pressure
  - muscle contractility
  - nerve impulse transmission
  - growth

Minerals may be classified as major minerals or trace minerals.

Major minerals

- Calcium
- Chloride
- Magnesium
- Phosphorus
- Potassium
- Sodium

Trace minerals

- Chromium
- Cobalt
- Copper
- Fluorine
- Iodine
- Iron
- Manganese
- Molybdenum
- Selenium
- Zinc

Guide to vitamins and minerals

Good health requires intake of adequate amounts of vitamins and minerals to meet the body's metabolic needs. A vitamin or mineral excess or deficiency can lead to various disorders. This chart reviews major functions of vitamins and minerals.

Vitamin or mineral	Major functions
Water-soluble vitamins	
Vitamin C (ascorbic acid)	Collagen production, fine bone and tooth formation, iodine conservation, healing, red blood cell (RBC) formation, infection resistance
Vitamin B_1 (thiamine)	Blood formation, carbohydrate metabolism, circulation, digestion, growth, learning ability, muscle tone maintenance, central nervous system (CNS) maintenance
Vitamin B_2 (riboflavin)	RBC formation; energy metabolism; cell respiration; epithelial, eye, and mucosal tissue maintenance
Vitamin B_6 (pyridoxine)	Antibody formation, digestion, deoxyribonucleic acid (DNA) and ribonucleic acid (RNA) synthesis, fat and protein utilization, amino acid metabolism, hemoglobin production, CNS maintenance
Folic acid (folacin, pteroylglutamic acid)	Cell growth and reproduction, digestion, liver function, DNA and RNA formation, protein metabolism, RBC formation
Niacin (nicotinic acid, nicotinamide, niacinamide)	Circulation, cholesterol level reduction, growth, hydrochloric acid production, metabolism (carbohydrate, protein, fat), sex hormone production
Vitamin B_{12} (cyanocobalamin)	RBC formation, cellular and nutrient metabolism, tissue growth, nerve cell maintenance, appetite stimulation
Fat-soluble vitamins	
Vitamin A	Body tissue repair and maintenance, infection resistance, bone growth, nervous system development, cell membrane metabolism and structure, night vision
Vitamin D (calciferol)	Calcium and phosphorus metabolism (bone formation), myocardial function, nervous system maintenance, normal blood clotting
Vitamin E (tocopherol)	Aging retardation, anticlotting factor, diuresis, fertility, lung protection (antipollution), male potency, muscle and nerve cell membrane maintenance, myocardial perfusion, serum cholesterol reduction
Vitamin K (menadione)	Liver synthesis of prothrombin and other blood-clotting factors

Continued!

Guide to vitamins and minerals *(continued)*

Vitamin or mineral	Major functions
Minerals	
Calcium	Blood clotting, bone and tooth formation, cardiac rhythm, cell membrane permeability, muscle growth and contraction, nerve impulse transmission
Chloride	Maintenance of fluid, electrolyte, acid-base, and osmotic pressure balance
Magnesium	Acid-base balance, metabolism, protein synthesis, muscle relaxation, cellular respiration, nerve impulse transmission
Phosphorus	Bone and tooth formation, cell growth and repair, energy production
Potassium	Cardiac rhythm, muscle contraction, nerve impulse transmission, rapid growth, fluid distribution and osmotic pressure balance, acid-base balance
Sodium	Cellular fluid-level maintenance, muscle contraction, acid-base balance, cell permeability, muscle function, nerve impulse transmission
Fluoride (fluorine)	Bone and tooth formation
Iodine	Thyroid hormone production, energy production, metabolism, physical and mental development
Iron	Growth (in children), hemoglobin production, stress and disease resistance, cellular respiration, oxygen transport
Selenium	Immune mechanisms, mitochondrial adenosine triphosphate synthesis, cellular protection
Zinc	Burn and wound healing, carbohydrate digestion, metabolism (carbohydrate, fat, protein), prostate gland function, reproductive organ growth and development, cell growth

Digestion and absorption

Nutrients are digested in the GI tract by enzymes that split large units into smaller ones—a process called *hydrolysis*.

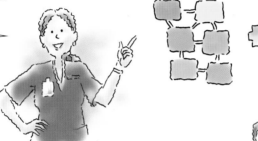

In hydrolysis, a compound unites with water and then splits into simpler compounds.

The smaller units are then absorbed from the small intestine and transported to the liver through the portal venous system.

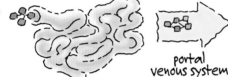

portal
venous system

Carbohydrate digestion and absorption

Digestion begins in the mouth and continues through the small intestines. After the nutrients are broken down, they're absorbed through the intestinal mucosa.

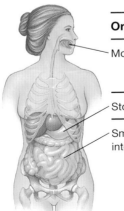

Organ	Action
Mouth	■ Chewing breaks down food into smaller particles. ■ The salivary enzyme amylase acts on starch to break it down first into dextrins and then into maltose.
Stomach	■ Peristalsis mixes food particles with gastric secretions.
Small intestine	■ The pancreatic enzyme amylase continues the breakdown of starch to maltose. ■ The intestinal enzyme sucrase acts on sucrose to produce fructose. ■ The intestinal enzyme lactase acts on lactose to produce galactose. ■ The intestinal enzyme maltase acts on maltose to produce glucose.

Protein digestion and absorption

Enzymes digest proteins by hydrolyzing the peptide bonds that link the amino acids of the protein chains.

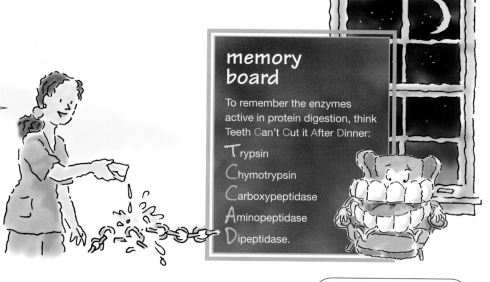

memory board

To remember the enzymes active in protein digestion, think Teeth Can't Cut it After Dinner:

Trypsin

Chymotrypsin

Carboxypeptidase

Aminopeptidase

Dipeptidase.

After the intestinal mucosal peptidases break down peptides into their constituent amino acids, they're absorbed through the intestinal mucosa by active transport mechanisms. They then travel to the liver, where any amino acids not needed for protein synthesis are converted into glucose.

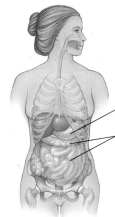

Enzymes active in protein digestion

Organ	Active enzymes	Digestive action
Stomach	Pepsin	Breaks protein into polypeptides
Intestine	Trypsin-pancreatic enzyme	Breaks protein and polypeptides into tripeptides and dipeptides
	Chymotrypsin-pancreatic enzyme	Breaks protein and polypeptides into tripeptides and dipeptides
	Carboxypeptidase	Breaks polypeptides into simpler peptides and amino acids
	Aminopeptidase	Breaks polypeptides into peptides, dipeptides, and amino acids
	Dipeptidase	Breaks dipeptides into amino acids

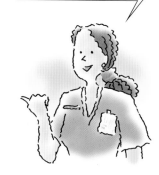

Fat digestion and absorption

Most fat digestion occurs in the small intestine.

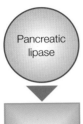

1 Pancreatic lipase breaks down fats and phospholipids into a mixture of:
■ glycerol
■ short-chain fatty acids
■ long-chain fatty acids
■ monoglycerides.

| Glycerol |
| Short-chain fatty acids |
| Long-chain fatty acids |
| Monoglycerides |

Pancreatic lipase

Fats, phospholipids

2 Because fat doesn't dissolve in water, it enters the duodenum in a congealed mass. To help with digestion, the gallbladder releases bile into the duodenum. Bile acts to *emulsify* the fat (disperse the fat into small droplets that can become suspended in the watery content of the digestive tract). This allows lipase to accelerate its digestion of the fat.

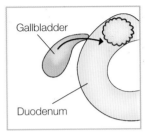

Gallbladder

Duodenum

Meanwhile, back in the small intestines...

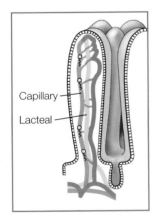

3 Absorption of fat occurs in the villi of the small intestines. Glycerol diffuses directly through the intestinal mucosa, whereas short-chain fatty acids are absorbed into the bloodstream via the intestinal capillaries. After they're in the bloodstream, they're carried to the liver via the portal venous system.

Capillary

Lacteal

4 Long-chain fatty acids and monoglycerides are too large to be absorbed by the capillaries. Therefore, they're absorbed into the fatty walls of the villi and changed into triglycerides. These triglycerides are then coated with cholesterol and protein, forming lipoprotein particles called *chylomicrons*.

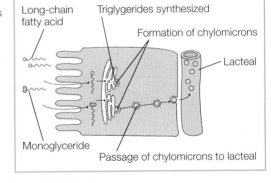

Long-chain fatty acid

Triglygerides synthesized

Formation of chylomicrons

Lacteal

Monoglyceride

Passage of chylomicrons to lacteal

The chylomicrons enter a lacteal, where they're carried through the lymphatic channels to the thoracic duct. From the thoracic duct, they enter the bloodstream and are distributed to body cells. In the cells, fats are extracted from the chylomicrons and broken down by enzymes into fatty acids and glycerol. Then they're absorbed and recombined in fat cells, reforming triglycerides for storage and later use.

Enzymes active in fat digestion

Organ	Active enzymes	Digestive action
Mouth	■ Lingual lipase	Minimal amount of fat digestion
Liver	■ Bile	Prepares fat for absorption by breaking it into tiny particles (emulsification)
Pancreas	■ Pancreatic lipase	Breaks down fats into fatty acids and glycerol

Metabolism

Through metabolism, food substances are transformed into energy or materials that the body can use or store. Metabolism involves two processes:
■ anabolism—synthesizing complex substances out of simpler ones
■ catabolism—breaking down complex substances into simpler ones or into energy.

Carbohydrate metabolism

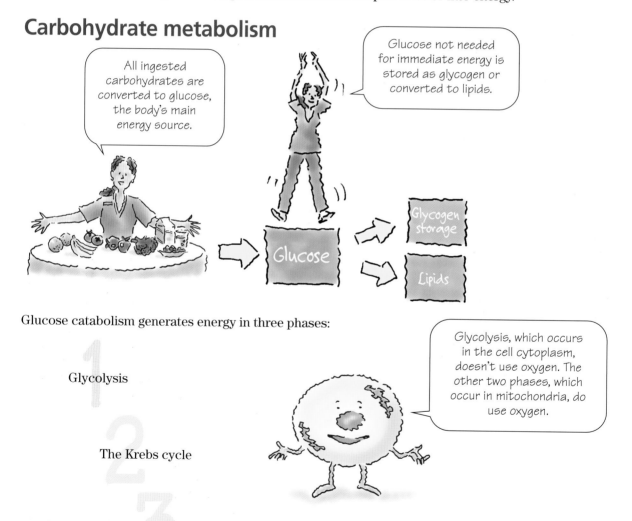

All ingested carbohydrates are converted to glucose, the body's main energy source.

Glucose not needed for immediate energy is stored as glycogen or converted to lipids.

Glucose

Glycogen storage

Lipids

Glucose catabolism generates energy in three phases:

1 Glycolysis

2 The Krebs cycle

3 The electron-transport chain

Glycolysis, which occurs in the cell cytoplasm, doesn't use oxygen. The other two phases, which occur in mitochondria, do use oxygen.

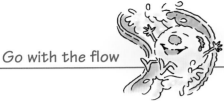

Go with the flow

Tracking the glucose pathway

Glycolysis

Glycolysis, the first phase, breaks apart one molecule of glucose to form pyruvate, which yields energy in the form of adenosine triphosphate (ATP) and acetyl coenzyme A (CoA).

Krebs cycle

The second phase, the Krebs cycle, continues carbohydrate metabolism. Fragments of acetyl CoA join to oxaloacetic acid to form citric acid. The CoA molecule breaks off from the acetyl group and may form more acetyl CoA molecules. Citric acid is first converted into intermediate compounds and then back into oxaloacetic acid. The Krebs cycle also liberates carbon dioxide (CO_2).

Electron-transport chain

In the third phase of glucose catabolism, molecules on the inner mitochondrial membrane attract electrons from hydrogen atoms and carry them through oxidation-reduction reactions in the mitochondria. The hydrogen ions produced in the Krebs cycle then combine with oxygen (O_2) to form water (H_2O).

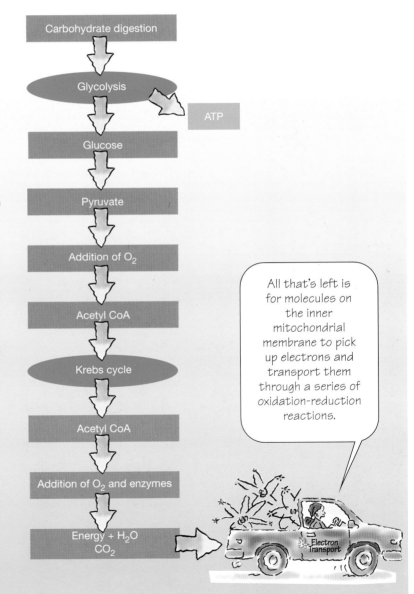

Carbohydrate digestion

Glycolysis

ATP

Glucose

Pyruvate

Addition of O_2

Acetyl CoA

Krebs cycle

Acetyl CoA

Addition of O_2 and enzymes

Energy + H_2O
CO_2

All that's left is for molecules on the inner mitochondrial membrane to pick up electrons and transport them through a series of oxidation-reduction reactions.

Electron Transport

Regulation of blood glucose levels

Because all ingested carbohydrates are converted to glucose, the body depends on certain organ systems to regulate blood glucose levels.

The role of the liver

When blood glucose levels exceed the body's immediate needs, hormones stimulate the liver to convert glucose into glycogen or lipids.

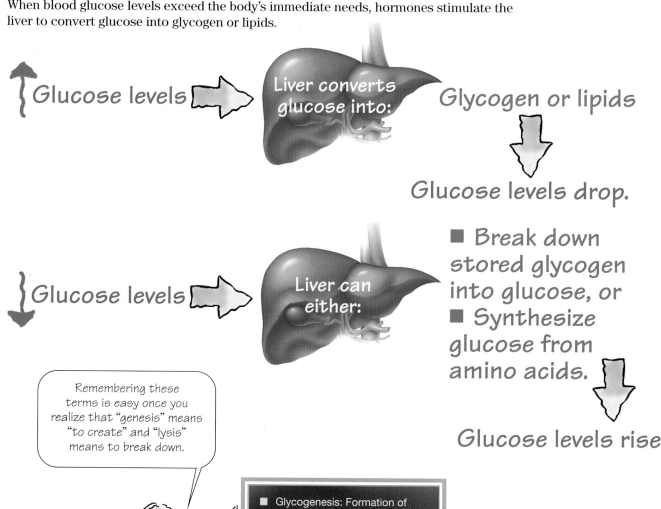

↑ Glucose levels ➡ Liver converts glucose into: Glycogen or lipids

Glucose levels drop.

↓ Glucose levels ➡ Liver can either: ■ Break down stored glycogen into glucose, or ■ Synthesize glucose from amino acids.

Glucose levels rise

Remembering these terms is easy once you realize that "genesis" means "to create" and "lysis" means to break down.

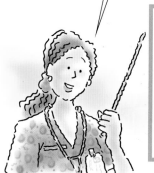

■ Glycogenesis: Formation of glycogen

■ Lipogenesis: Formation of lipids

■ Glycogenolysis: Breakdown of glycogen to glucose

■ Gluconeogenesis: Synthesis of glucose from amino acids

The role of muscles

During vigorous muscular activity, when oxygen requirements exceed the oxygen supply, muscle cells break down glycogen to yield lactic acid and energy. Lactic acid then builds up in the muscles, and muscle glycogen is depleted.

> Muscle cells can convert glucose to glycogen for storage. However, they lack the enzymes needed to convert glycogen back to glucose.

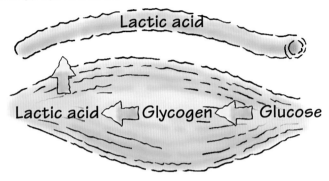

Some of the lactic acid diffuses from muscle cells, is transported to the liver, and is reconverted to glycogen. The liver converts the newly formed glycogen to glucose, which travels through the bloodstream to the muscles and reforms into glycogen.

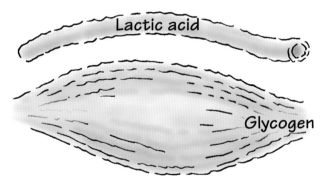
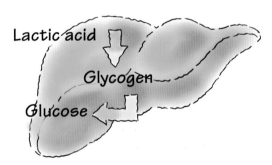

When muscle exertion stops, some of the accumulated lactic acid converts back to pyruvic acid. Pyruvic acid is oxidized completely to yield energy by means of the Krebs cycle and electron-transport system.

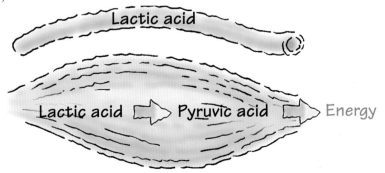

The role of hormones

Hormones regulate blood glucose levels by stimulating certain metabolic processes. Insulin, produced by the pancreatic islet cells, is the only hormone that significantly reduces blood glucose levels. In addition to promoting cell uptake and use of glucose as an energy source, insulin promotes glucose storage as glycogen (glycogenesis) and lipids (lipogenesis).

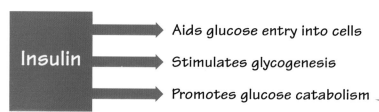

How insulin affects blood glucose level

Insulin
- Aids glucose entry into cells
- Stimulates glycogenesis
- Promotes glucose catabolism

Decreased blood glucose level

Protein metabolism

Proteins are absorbed as amino acids and carried by the portal venous system to the liver and then throughout the body by blood. Absorbed amino acids mix with other amino acids in the body's amino acid pool. These other amino acids may either be synthesized by the body from other substances (such as keto acids) or produced by protein breakdown. The body can't store amino acids. Instead, it converts them to protein or glucose or catabolizes them to provide energy.

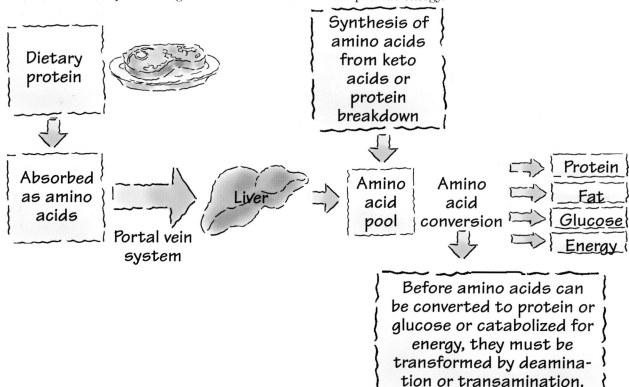

Dietary protein

Absorbed as amino acids

Portal vein system

Liver

Synthesis of amino acids from keto acids or protein breakdown

Amino acid pool

Amino acid conversion
- Protein
- Fat
- Glucose
- Energy

Before amino acids can be converted to protein or glucose or catabolized for energy, they must be transformed by deamination or transamination.

Deamination

- This occurs when an amino group ($-NH_2$) splits off from an amino acid molecule.
- A molecule of ammonia and one of keto acid are formed as a result.
- Most of the ammonia is converted to urea and excreted in the urine.

Transamination

- This occurs when the amino acid is converted to a keto acid.
- The original keto acid is then converted to an amino acid.

Essential and nonessential amino acids

Amino acids are the structural units of proteins. They're classified as essential or nonessential based on whether the human body can synthesize them.

These amino acids can't be synthesized and must be obtained from the diet.

The body can synthesize these amino acids. While they're needed for protein synthesis, they're nonessential in the diet.

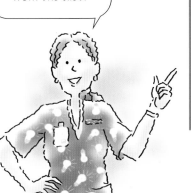

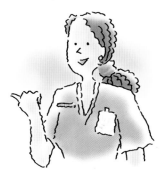

Essential	Nonessential
■ Histidine	■ Alanine
■ Isoleucine	■ Arginine
■ Leucine	■ Asparagine
■ Lysine	■ Aspartic acid
■ Methionine	■ Cystine
■ Phenylalanine	■ Glutamic acid
■ Threonine	■ Glycine
■ Tryptophan	■ Hydroxyproline
■ Valine	■ Proline
	■ Serine
	■ Tyrosine

Lipid metabolism

Until required for use as fuel, lipids are stored in adipose tissue within cells. When needed for energy, each fat molecule is hydrolyzed to glycerol and three molecules of fatty acids. Glycerol can be converted to pyruvic acid and then to acetyl CoA, which enters the Krebs cycle.

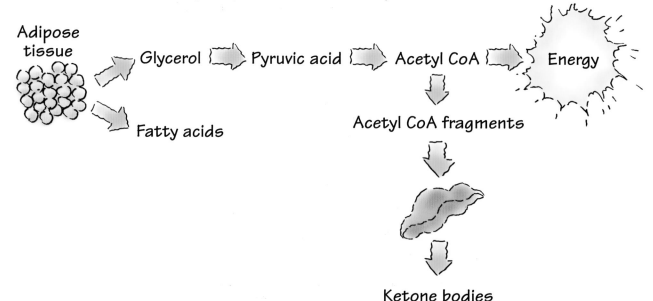

Leftovers

The liver normally forms ketone bodies from acetyl CoA fragments, derived largely from fatty acid catabolism. Acetyl CoA molecules yield three types of ketone bodies:

1 Acetoacetic acid
  ■ Results from the combination of two acetyl CoA molecules and subsequent release of CoA from these molecules
2 Beta-hydroxybutyric acid
  ■ Forms when hydrogen is added to the oxygen atom in the acetoacetic acid molecule
  ■ Term "beta" indicates the location of the carbon atom containing the OH group
3 Acetone
  ■ Forms when the COOH group of acetoacetic acid releases carbon dioxide
  ■ Oxidized by muscle, brain, and other tissues for energy

Too much of a good thing

When the supply of glucose for energy is inadequate—such as from fasting, starvation, or uncontrolled diabetes (in which the body can't break down glucose)—the body must switch to fat as its primary energy source. This results in an excess production of ketone bodies. The accumulation of ketone bodies lowers the body's pH, disturbing normal acid-base balance and leading to ketosis.

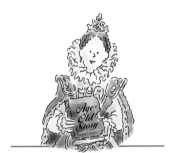

Age-old story

Age-related nutrition changes

Caloric needs decrease with age, but protein, vitamin, and mineral requirements usually remain the same throughout life. The body's ability to process these nutrients, however, is affected by the aging process. Listed here are physiologic changes related to aging along with their effects on nutrition:

- Diminished intestinal motility > Constipation
- Decreased renal function > Susceptibility to dehydration and formation of renal calculi
- Impaired mobility > Loss of calcium and nitrogen
- Reduced pepsin and hydrochloric acid secretion > Diminished absorption of calcium and vitamins B_1 and B_2
- Decreased salivary flow and diminished sense of taste > Decreased appetite
- Thinning of tooth enamel > Brittle teeth
- Decreased biting force > Difficulty chewing
- Diminished gag reflex > Choking

VISION QUEST

Rebus riddle

Sound out each group of symbols and letters to reveal information about one of the body's main nutrients.

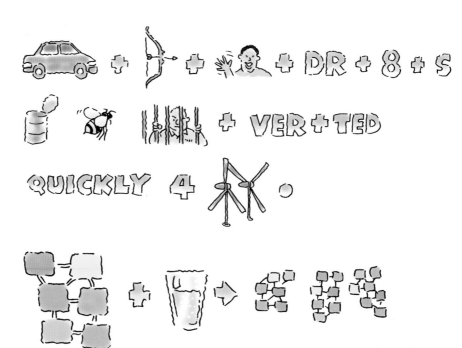

Show and tell

Using the illustrations as a guide, describe two processes by which nutrients are digested and then absorbed.

1. _____
_____
_____

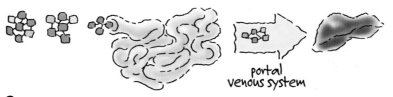

portal venous system

2. _____
_____
_____

Answers: Rebus riddle Carbohydrates can be converted quickly for energy. Show and tell 1. In hydrolysis, a compound unites with water and then splits into simpler compounds. 2. The smaller units are then absorbed from the small intestine and transported to the liver through the portal venous system.

15
Urinary system

- Components of the urinary system 192
- Urine formation 197
- Hormones and the urinary system 198
- Vision quest 200

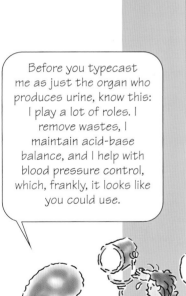

Before you typecast me as just the organ who produces urine, know this: I play a lot of roles. I remove wastes, I maintain acid-base balance, and I help with blood pressure control, which, frankly, it looks like you could use.

Components of the urinary system

The urinary system consists of two kidneys, two ureters, the bladder, and the urethra.

The right kidney extends slightly lower than the left because of the space taken up by the liver. Consequently, the right ureter is slightly shorter than the left one.

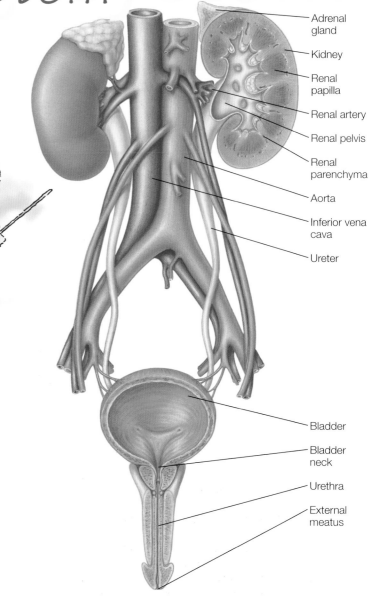

- Adrenal gland
- Kidney
- Renal papilla
- Renal artery
- Renal pelvis
- Renal parenchyma
- Aorta
- Inferior vena cava
- Ureter
- Bladder
- Bladder neck
- Urethra
- External meatus

Kidneys

The kidneys are bean-shaped, highly vascular organs. They form urine to remove waste from the body, maintain acid-base and fluid-electrolyte balance, and assist in blood pressure control.

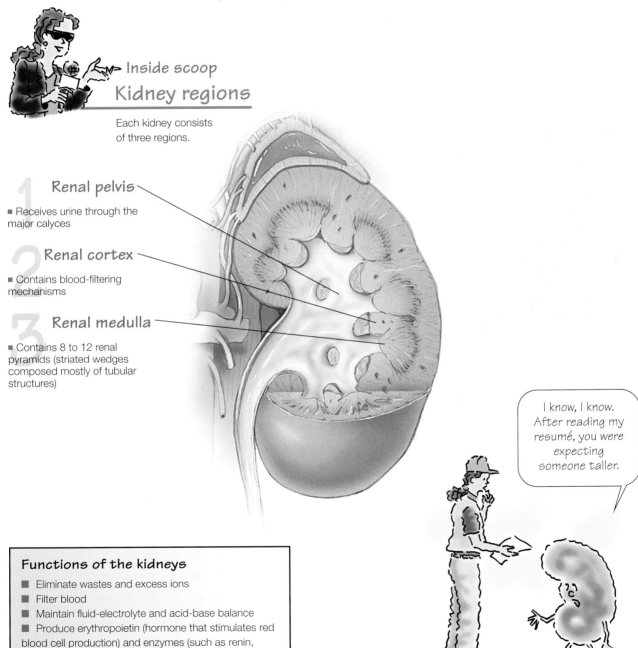

M→ Inside scoop
Kidney regions

Each kidney consists of three regions.

1
Renal pelvis
■ Receives urine through the major calyces

2
Renal cortex
■ Contains blood-filtering mechanisms

3
Renal medulla
■ Contains 8 to 12 renal pyramids (striated wedges composed mostly of tubular structures)

I know, I know. After reading my resumé, you were expecting someone taller.

Functions of the kidneys

■ Eliminate wastes and excess ions
■ Filter blood
■ Maintain fluid-electrolyte and acid-base balance
■ Produce erythropoietin (hormone that stimulates red blood cell production) and enzymes (such as renin, which governs blood pressure and kidney function)
■ Convert vitamin D to a more active form

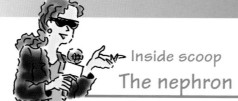

Inside scoop
The nephron

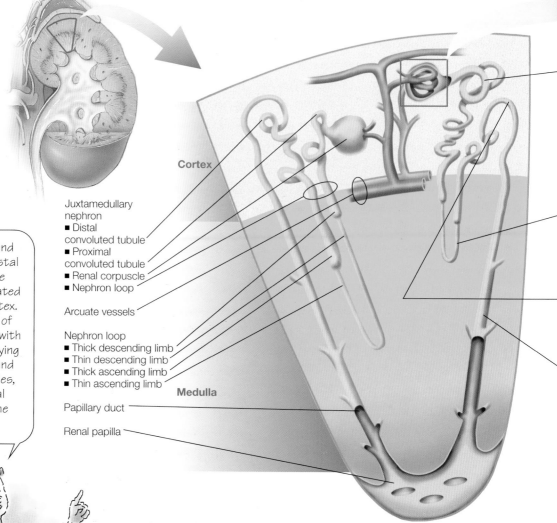

Cortex

Juxtamedullary
nephron
■ Distal
convoluted tubule
■ Proximal
convoluted tubule
■ Renal corpuscle
■ Nephron loop

Arcuate vessels

Nephron loop
■ Thick descending limb
■ Thin descending limb
■ Thick ascending limb
■ Thin ascending limb

Medulla

Papillary duct

Renal papilla

The glomeruli and proximal and distal tubules of the nephron are located in the renal cortex. The long loops of Henle, together with their accompanying blood vessels and collecting tubules, form the renal pyramids in the medulla.

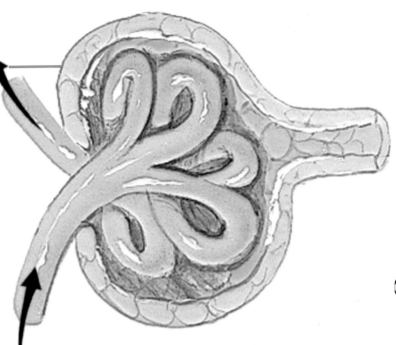

The nephron is the kidney's basic functional unit and the site of urine formation.

1 The **proximal convoluted tubule** circulates water and reabsorbs nearly all the glucose, amino acids, metabolites, and electrolytes from the filtrate into nearby capillaries.

2 The **loop of Henle** concentrates the filtrate through electrolyte exchange and reabsorption to produce a hyperosmolar fluid.

3 The **distal convoluted tubule** is the point where filtrate enters the collecting tubule; here, sodium is reabsorbed under the influence of aldosterone.

4 The **collecting tubule** is the distal end of the nephron and provides the site of final concentration.

Renal corpuscle

Known as the beginning of the nephron, the renal corpuscle consists of the glomerulus (a cluster of capillaries) and Bowman's capsule (surrounds the glomerulus and collects filtrate). Unfiltered blood flows into the glomerulus through the afferent arteriole. After being filtered by the glomerulus, it flows out through the efferent arteriole and into the proximal convoluted tubule.

Functions of the nephron

■ Filters fluids, wastes, electrolytes, acids, and bases into the tubular system
■ Selectively reabsorbs and secretes ions

Age-old story

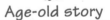

Age-related urinary system changes

■ Diminished kidney function (begins at age 40; by age 90, may decrease by 50%)
■ Decreased glomerular filtration rate (due to changes in kidney vasculature)
■ Decreased kidney blood flow (due to reduced cardiac output and atherosclerotic changes)
■ Decline in tubular reabsorption and renal concentrating ability (due to a decrease in the size and number of functioning nephrons)
■ Tendency to develop bladder infections (due to chronic urine retention from weakened bladder muscles)
■ Impaired renal clearance of drugs
■ Reduced bladder size and capacity
■ Decreased renal ability to respond to variations in sodium intake
■ Increased blood urea nitrogen levels

Ureters, bladder, and urethra

The **URETERS** are fibromuscular tubes that connect each kidney to the bladder. They act as conduits that carry urine from the kidneys to the bladder. The left ureter is usually slightly longer than the right ureter (because the left kidney sits higher than the right).

The **BLADDER** is a hollow, sphere-shaped, muscular organ in the pelvis. Its function is to store urine. (The normal adult bladder capacity ranges from 500 to 600 ml.)

The base of the bladder contains three openings that form a triangular area called the **TRIGONE**. Two of the openings connect the bladder to the ureters, and the third connects the bladder to the urethra.

The **URETHRA** is a small duct that channels urine from the bladder out of the body. In the female, the urethra is embedded in the anterior wall of the vagina behind the symphysis pubis. In the male, the urethra passes vertically through the prostate gland and then extends through the urogenital diaphragm and the penis.

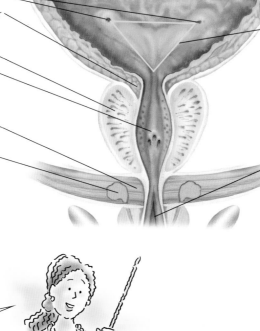

Cut edge of peritoneum

Smooth muscle

Rugae

Opening of ureter

Internal urinary sphincter

Prostate gland

Prostatic urethra

External urinary sphincter

Bulbourethral gland

Although the kidneys juggle a lot of the urinary system's responsibility, other structures also play key roles. This illustration shows these structures in a male.

Urine formation

Urine formation is one of the main functions of the urinary system. Urine formation results from three processes that occur in the nephrons: glomerular filtration, tubular reabsorption, and tubular secretion.

How the kidneys form urine

STEP 1
Glomerular filtration

As blood flows into the glomerulus, filtration occurs. In glomerular filtration, active transport from the proximal convoluted tubules leads to reabsorption of sodium (Na^+) and glucose into nearby circulation. Osmosis then causes water (H_2O) reabsorption.

STEP 2
Tubular reabsorption

In tubular reabsorption, a substance moves from the filtrate back from the distal convoluted tubules, into the peritubular capillaries. Active transport results in Na^+ reabsorption. The presence of antidiuretic hormone causes H_2O reabsorption.

STEP 3
Tubular secretion

In tubular secretion, a substance moves from the peritubular capillaries into the tubular filtrate. Peritubular capillaries then secrete ammonia (NH_3) and hydrogen (H^+).

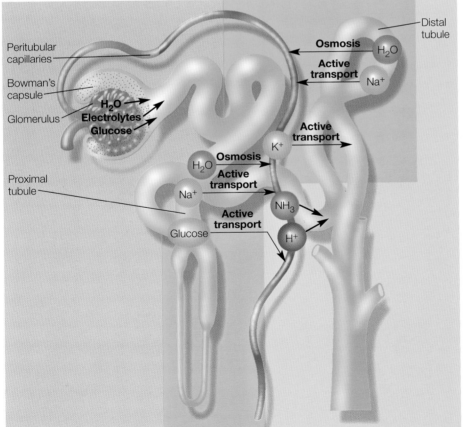

Peritubular capillaries

Bowman's capsule

Glomerulus

H_2O
Electrolytes
Glucose

Proximal tubule

Osmosis
H_2O
Active transport
Na^+

Glucose

Active transport

Osmosis
Active transport

K^+

Active transport

NH_3

H^+

Distal tubule

Osmosis
H_2O
Active transport
Na^+

Active transport

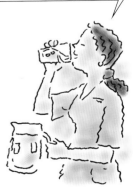

Total daily urine output averages 720 to 2,400 ml. However, that varies with fluid intake and climate. For example, after drinking a large volume of fluid, urine output increases as the body rapidly excretes excess water. If a person restricts water intake, has an excessive intake of sodium, or perspires heavily, urine output decreases as the body retains water to restore normal fluid concentration.

Hormones and the urinary system

A diuretic increases the rate of urine formation. So, an anti-diuretic—as in antidiuretic hormone—decreases the rate of urine formation.

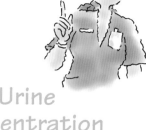

Hormones play a major role in the urinary system, including helping the body to manage tubular reabsorption and secretion.

Antidiuretic hormone

Antidiuretic hormone (ADH) regulates levels of urine output.

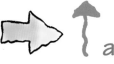 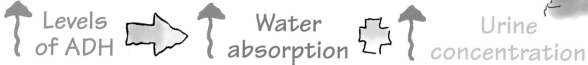

↑ Levels of ADH ➡ ↑ Water absorption ✚ ↑ Urine concentration

↓ Levels of ADH ➡ ↓ Water absorption ✚ ↓ Urine concentration

How ADH works

Low blood volume and increased serum osmolality are sensed by the hypothalamus, which signals the pituitary gland.

The pituitary gland secretes ADH into the bloodstream.

ADH causes the kidneys to retain water.

Water retention boosts blood volume and decreases serum osmolality.

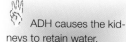

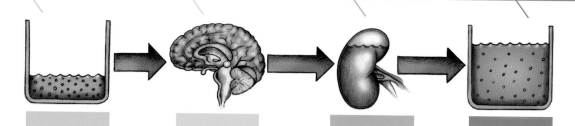

Renin-angiotensin-aldosterone system

The renin-angiotensin-aldosterone system regulates the body's sodium and water levels and blood pressure.

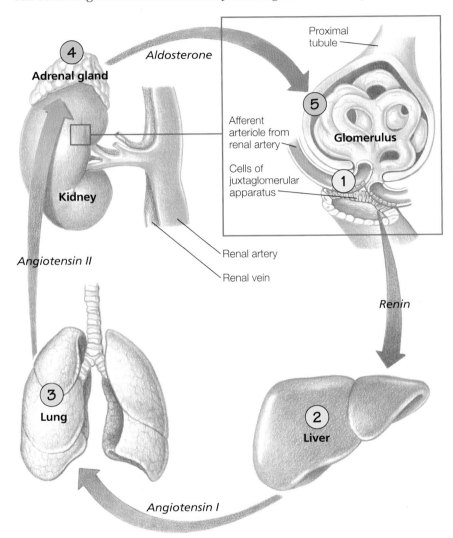

4 Adrenal gland

Aldosterone

Proximal tubule

5

Afferent arteriole from renal artery

Cells of juxtaglomerular apparatus

Glomerulus

1

Kidney

Renal artery

Renal vein

Angiotensin II

Renin

3

Lung

2

Liver

Angiotensin I

1 Juxtaglomerular cells near the glomeruli in each kidney secrete the enzyme renin into the blood.

2 Renin circulates throughout the body and converts angiotensinogen, made in the liver, into angiotensin I.

3 In the lungs, angiotensin I is converted by hydrolysis to angiotensin II.

4 Angiotensin II acts on the adrenal cortex to stimulate production of the hormone aldosterone.

5 Aldosterone acts on the juxtaglomerular cells to increase sodium and water retention and to stimulate or depress further renin secretion, completing the feedback system that automatically readjusts homeostasis.

VISION QUEST

Able to label?

Identify the key structures of the urinary system shown in this illustration.

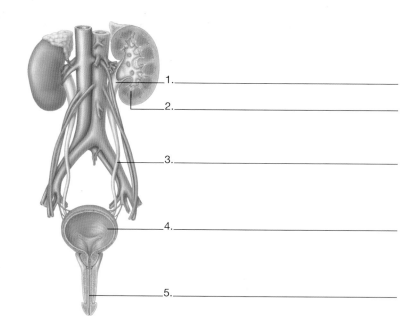

1. _____
2. _____
3. _____
4. _____
5. _____

Show and tell

Using the illustration provided as a guide, describe how ADH regulates fluid balance.

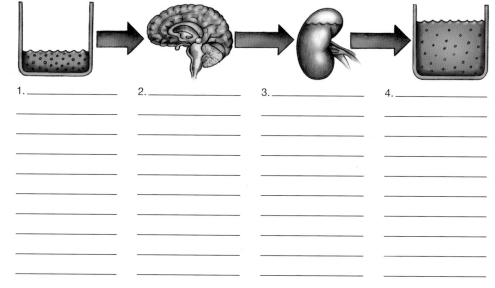

1. _____
_____
_____
_____
_____
_____
_____
_____

2. _____
_____
_____
_____
_____
_____
_____
_____

3. _____
_____
_____
_____
_____
_____
_____
_____

4. _____
_____
_____
_____
_____
_____
_____
_____

Answers: Able to label? 1. Ureter, 2. Renal pelvis, 3. Ureter, 4. Bladder, 5.Urethra Show and tell: 1. Low blood volume and increased serum osmolality are sensed by the hypothalamus, which signals the pituitary gland. 2. The pituitary gland secretes ADH into the bloodstream. 3. ADH causes the kidneys to retain water. 4. Water retention boosts blood volume and decreases serum osmolality.

16
Fluids, electrolytes, acids, and bases

● Fluid balance 202
● Electrolyte balance 209
● Acid-base balance 211
● Vision quest 212

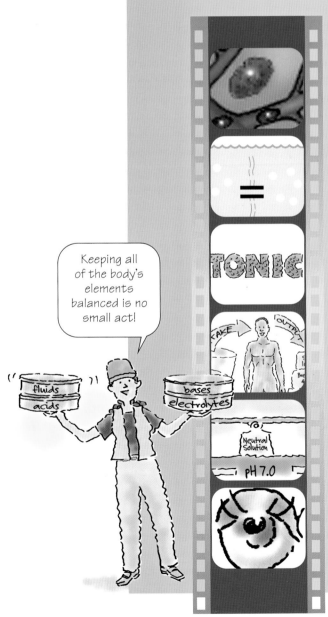

Keeping all of the body's elements balanced is no small act!

Fluid balance

Each day, the body takes in fluid through the GI tract—from foods and liquids as well as from the oxidation of food—and loses it in the form of urine and stool and through the skin and lungs.

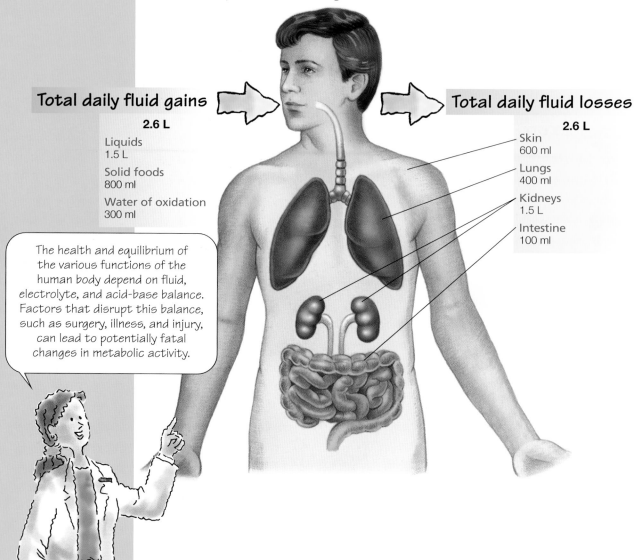

Total daily fluid gains

2.6 L

Liquids
1.5 L

Solid foods
800 ml

Water of oxidation
300 ml

Total daily fluid losses

2.6 L

Skin
600 ml

Lungs
400 ml

Kidneys
1.5 L

Intestine
100 ml

The health and equilibrium of the various functions of the human body depend on fluid, electrolyte, and acid-base balance. Factors that disrupt this balance, such as surgery, illness, and injury, can lead to potentially fatal changes in metabolic activity.

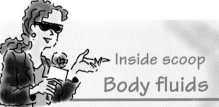

Inside scoop
Body fluids

The body contains four types of fluids.

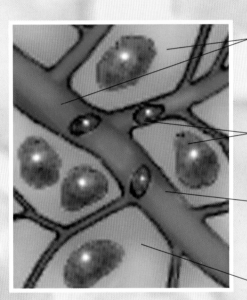

1 ECF

Extracellular fluid (ECF) is found in the spaces between the cells and includes interstitial fluid (ISF) and intravascular fluid (IVF).

2 ICF

Intracellular fluid (ICF) is found within the individual cells of the body.

3 IVF

IVF is found within the plasma and the lymphatic system.

4 ISF

ISF is found in the loose tissue around cells.

Water weight

Water in the body exists in two major compartments that are separated by capillary walls and cell membranes. About two-thirds of the body's water is found within cells as ICF; the other one-third remains outside cells as ECF.

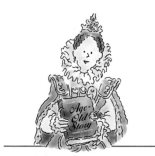

ECF accounts for approximately 20% of body weight, or approximately 14 L.		
IVF accounts for approximately 5% of body weight, or approximately 3.5 L.	**ISF** accounts for approximately 15% of body weight, or approximately 10.5 L.	
ICF accounts for approximately 40% of body weight, or approximately 28 L.		

memory board

To help remember which fluid belongs to which compartment, keep in mind the following:
- inter means **BETWEEN** (as in "interval")
- intra means **WITHIN** or inside (as in "intravenous").

Age-old story

Age-related fluid changes

The risk of suffering a fluid imbalance increases with age. Skeletal muscle mass declines, and the proportion of fat within the body increases. After age 60, water content drops to about 45%.

Likewise, the distribution of fluid within the body changes with age. For instance, about 15% of a typical young adult's total body weight is made up of ISF. That percentage progressively decreases with age.

Fluid forms and movement

Fluids in the body generally aren't found in pure forms. They're most commonly found in three different types of solutions: isotonic, hypotonic, and hypertonic.

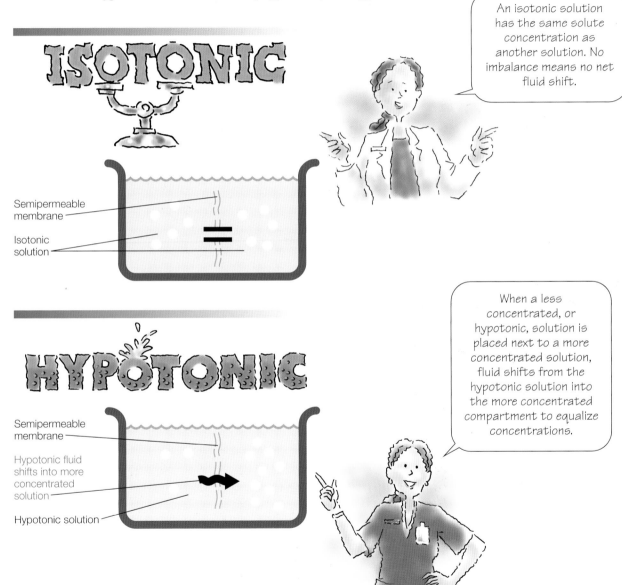

An isotonic solution has the same solute concentration as another solution. No imbalance means no net fluid shift.

ISOTONIC

Semipermeable membrane

Isotonic solution

When a less concentrated, or hypotonic, solution is placed next to a more concentrated solution, fluid shifts from the hypotonic solution into the more concentrated compartment to equalize concentrations.

HYPOTONIC

Semipermeable membrane

Hypotonic fluid shifts into more concentrated solution

Hypotonic solution

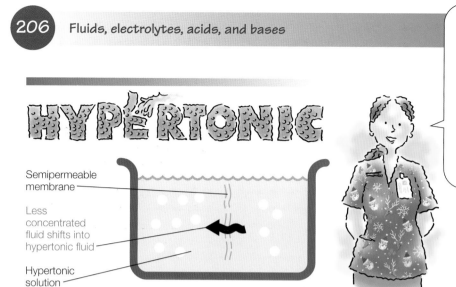

If one solution has more solutes than an adjacent solution, it has less fluid relative to the adjacent solution. Fluid will move out of the less concentrated solution into the more concentrated, or hypertonic, solution until both solutions have the same amount of solutes and fluid.

Semipermeable membrane

Less concentrated fluid shifts into hypertonic fluid

Hypertonic solution

Fluid movement within cells

Fluids and solutes move constantly within the body. That movement allows the body to maintain homeostasis, the constant state of balance the body seeks.

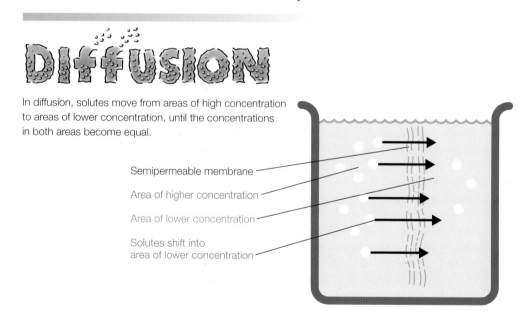

In diffusion, solutes move from areas of high concentration to areas of lower concentration, until the concentrations in both areas become equal.

Semipermeable membrane

Area of higher concentration

Area of lower concentration

Solutes shift into area of lower concentration

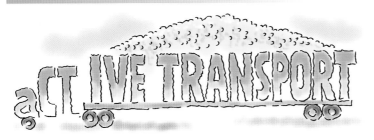

In active transport, solutes move from an area of lower concentration to an area of higher concentration.

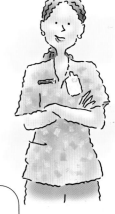

It takes energy to "go against the flow." In the case of active transport, moving against the concentration gradient uses energy in the form of adenosine triphosphate, or ATP.

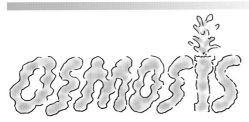

Semipermeable membrane

Area of higher concentration

Area of lower concentration

Energy from ATP pushes against the concentration gradient

Solute

ATP

Remember, in osmosis, *fluid* moves; in diffusion, *solutes* move.

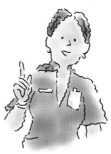

In osmosis, fluid moves passively from areas with more fluid (and fewer solutes) to areas with less fluid (and more solutes).

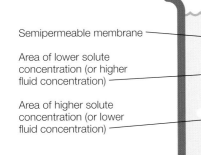

Semipermeable membrane

Area of lower solute concentration (or higher fluid concentration)

Area of higher solute concentration (or lower fluid concentration)

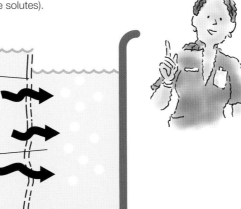

Fluid intake and output

Water normally enters the body from the GI tract through consumed liquids and solid foods, which may contain up to 97% water. Also, oxidation of food in the body yields carbon dioxide and about 300 ml of water (water of oxidation).

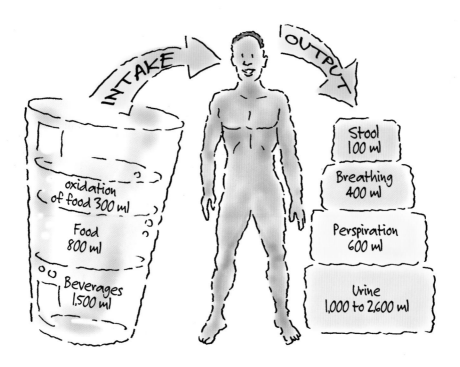

Electrolyte balance

Electrolytes are substances that break up into ions (electrically charged particles) when dissolved in water. To function normally, the body requires adequate amounts of each major electrolyte as well as a proper balance among the electrolytes.

> Normally, the electrical charges of cations balance the electrical charges of anions, keeping body fluids electrically neutral.

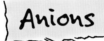

Anions
- Bicarbonate
- Chloride
- Phosphorus

Cations
- Calcium
- Magnesium
- Potassium
- Sodium

Electrolyte composition in ICF and ECF

Ions exist in low concentrations in body fluids. Because ICF and ECF cells are permeable to different substances, these compartments normally have different electrolyte compositions.

Electrolyte	ICF	ECF
Sodium	10 mEq/L	136 to 146 mEq/L
Potassium	140 mEq/L	3.6 to 5 mEq/L
Calcium	10 mEq/L	4.5 to 5.8 mEq/L
Magnesium	40 mEq/L	1.6 to 2.2 mEq/L
Chloride	4 mEq/L	96 to 106 mEq/L
Bicarbonate	10 mEq/L	24 to 28 mEq/L
Phosphate	100 mEq/L	1 to 1.5 mEq/L

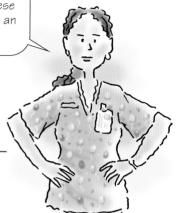

> Numerous mechanisms within the body help maintain electrolyte balance. Dysfunction or interruption of any of these mechanisms can produce an electrolyte imbalance.

Electrolytes profoundly affect the body's:
- water distribution
- osmolarity
- acid-base balance.

Go with the flow

Osmotic regulation of sodium and water

Serum sodium level decreases (water excess).
Serum osmolality drops to less than 280 mOsm/kg.
Thirst decreases, leading to diminished water intake.
Antidiuretic hormone (ADH) release is suppressed.
Renal water excretion increases.

Serum sodium increases (water deficit).
Serum osmolality increases to more than 300 mOsm/kg.
Thirst increases, leading to greater water intake.
ADH release increases.
Renal water excretion decreases.

Serum osmolality normalizes.

Acid-base balance

Physiologic survival requires *acid-base balance*, a stable concentration of hydrogen ions in body fluids. The degree of acidity or alkalinity of a solution is commonly expressed as pH, which refers to the concentration of hydrogen ions in a solution.

A neutral solution contains equal amounts of hydrogen (H⁺) and hydroxide (OH⁻) ions. A pH of 7 indicates neutrality.

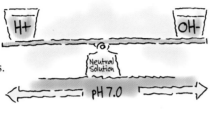

An acidic solution contains more hydrogen ions than hydroxide ions; its pH is less than 7.

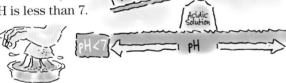

An alkaline, or basic, solution contains more hydroxide ions than hydrogen ions; its pH exceeds 7.

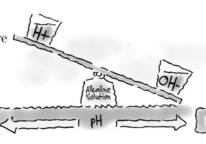

Acidic / Neutral / Basic (alkaline)	pH	Examples
	0	Hydrochloric acid
	1	Stomach acid
	2	Lemon juice
	3	Vinegar, cola, beer
	4	Tomatoes
	5	Black coffee
	6	Urine
	6.5	Saliva
	7	Distilled water, ICF
	7.4	Arterial blood
	8	Sea water
	9	Baking soda
	10.0	Great Salt Lake
	11	Household ammonia
	12	Bicarbonate of soda
	13	Oven cleaner
	14	Sodium hydroxide

The body maintains its acid-base balance within a narrow range by buffer systems and the lungs and kidneys, which neutralize and eliminate acids as rapidly as they're formed.

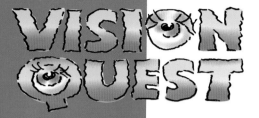

Matchmaker

Match the types of body fluids with their locations in the body, shown on the right.

A. ICF _____
B. IVF _____
C. ISF _____
D. ECF _____

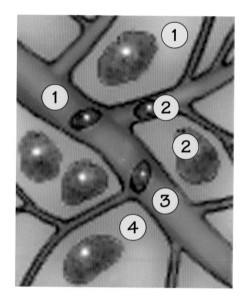

Show and tell

Using the illustration as a guide, describe the process of active transport.

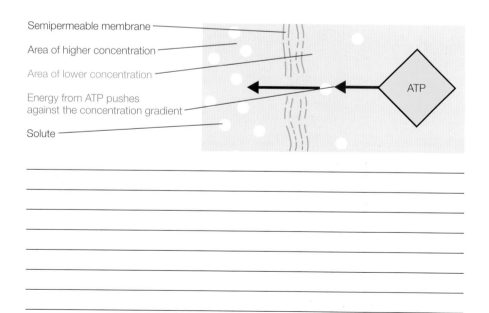

Semipermeable membrane

Area of higher concentration

Area of lower concentration

Energy from ATP pushes against the concentration gradient

Solute

ATP

_____

_____

_____

_____

_____

_____

_____

_____

17
Reproductive system

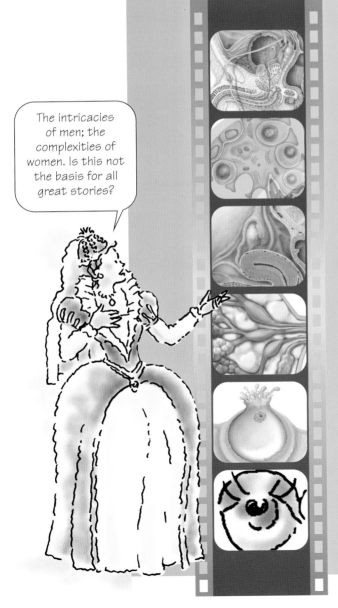

The intricacies of men; the complexities of women. Is this not the basis for all great stories?

■ Male reproductive system 214

■ Female reproductive system 219

■ Vision quest 224

Male reproductive system

The male reproductive system consists of the organs that produce, transfer, and introduce mature sperm into the female reproductive tract, where fertilization occurs.

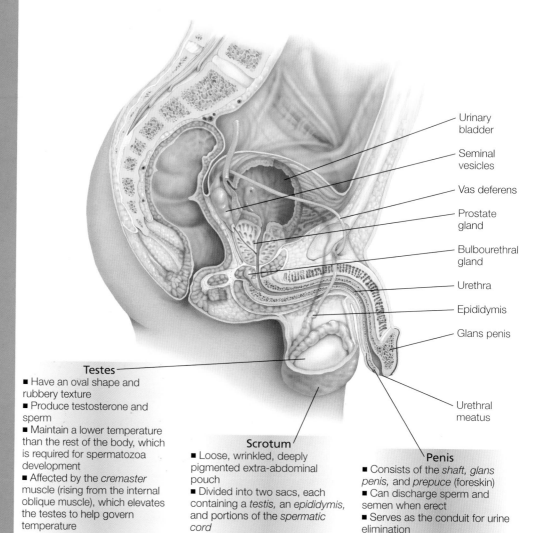

Urinary bladder

Seminal vesicles

Vas deferens

Prostate gland

Bulbourethral gland

Urethra

Epididymis

Glans penis

Urethral meatus

Testes
- Have an oval shape and rubbery texture
- Produce testosterone and sperm
- Maintain a lower temperature than the rest of the body, which is required for spermatozoa development
- Affected by the *cremaster* muscle (rising from the internal oblique muscle), which elevates the testes to help govern temperature

Scrotum
- Loose, wrinkled, deeply pigmented extra-abdominal pouch
- Divided into two sacs, each containing a *testis,* an *epididymis,* and portions of the *spermatic cord*

Penis
- Consists of the *shaft, glans penis,* and *prepuce* (foreskin)
- Can discharge sperm and semen when erect
- Serves as the conduit for urine elimination

Duct system

The male reproductive duct system conveys sperm from the testes to the ejaculatory ducts near the bladder.

Inside scoop
The testes

Each testis is encased by a dense white fibrous capsule called the *tunica albuginea.* This capsule enters the gland and sends out septa that divide the testis into more than 200 cone-shaped lobules.

Each lobule of the testis contains interstitial cells and seminiferous tubules. The seminiferous tubules are coiled and measure about 29½" (75 cm) unraveled. The tubules form a plexus called the *rete testis.* Efferent ductules, or sperm ducts, drain the rete testis and enter the tunica albuginea.

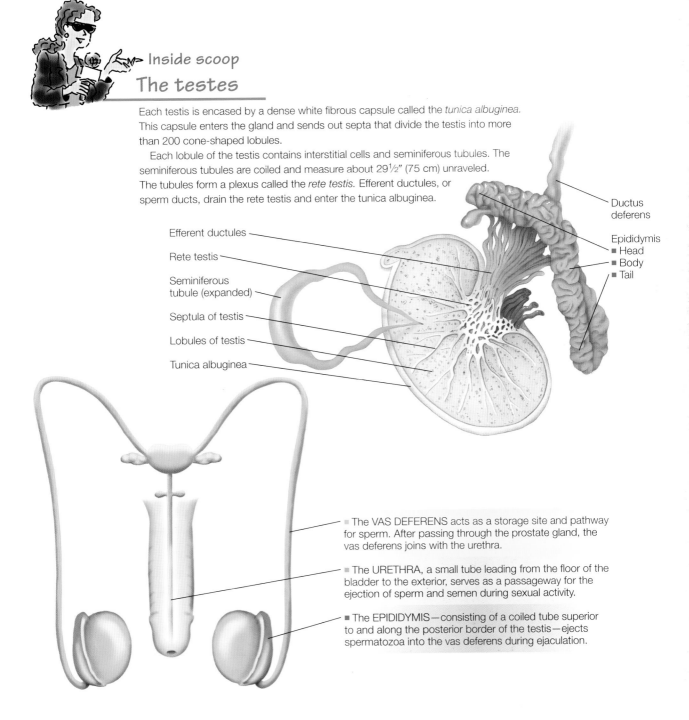

Efferent ductules

Rete testis

Seminiferous tubule (expanded)

Septula of testis

Lobules of testis

Tunica albuginea

Ductus deferens

Epididymis
■ Head
■ Body
■ Tail

■ The VAS DEFERENS acts as a storage site and pathway for sperm. After passing through the prostate gland, the vas deferens joins with the urethra.

■ The URETHRA, a small tube leading from the floor of the bladder to the exterior, serves as a passageway for the ejection of sperm and semen during sexual activity.

■ The EPIDIDYMIS—consisting of a coiled tube superior to and along the posterior border of the testis—ejects spermatozoa into the vas deferens during ejaculation.

Accessory reproductive glands

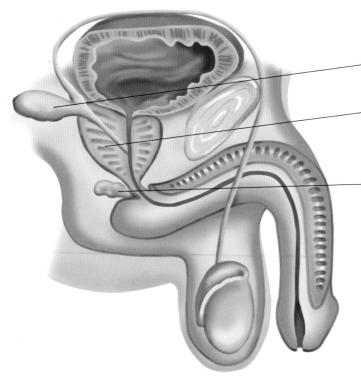

- The SEMINAL VESICLES—paired sacs at the base of the bladder—produce roughly 60% of the fluid portion of the semen.

- The PROSTATE GLAND—a walnut-size gland lying under the bladder and surrounding the urethra—produces about 30% of the fluid portion of semen. It continuously secretes prostatic fluid, a thin, milky, alkaline fluid that adds volume to the semen and enhances sperm motility.

- The BULBOURETHRAL GLANDS (also called *Cowper's glands*) are also paired glands and lie inferior to the prostate. They secrete an alkaline fluid that's important for counteracting the acid present in the male urethra and the female vagina. Mucus produced by these glands lubricates the urethra.

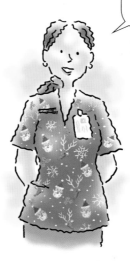

The accessory glands produce most of the semen.

Spermatogenesis

Sperm formation, or spermatogenesis, begins when a male reaches puberty and normally continues throughout life. It occurs in four stages.

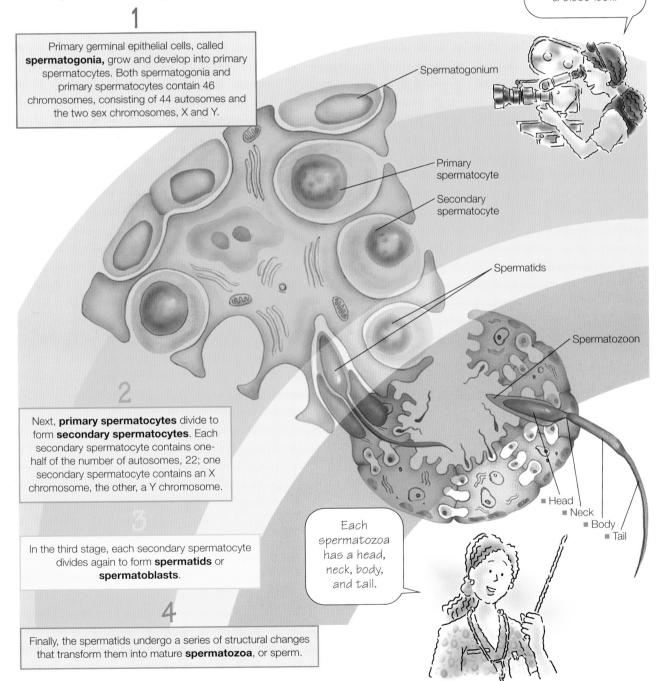

Deep inside the testes, sperm are being formed. Let's zoom in for a close look.

1

Primary germinal epithelial cells, called **spermatogonia,** grow and develop into primary spermatocytes. Both spermatogonia and primary spermatocytes contain 46 chromosomes, consisting of 44 autosomes and the two sex chromosomes, X and Y.

Spermatogonium

Primary spermatocyte

Secondary spermatocyte

Spermatids

Spermatozoon

2

Next, **primary spermatocytes** divide to form **secondary spermatocytes**. Each secondary spermatocyte contains one-half of the number of autosomes, 22; one secondary spermatocyte contains an X chromosome, the other, a Y chromosome.

■ Head
■ Neck
■ Body
■ Tail

3

In the third stage, each secondary spermatocyte divides again to form **spermatids** or **spermatoblasts**.

Each spermatozoa has a head, neck, body, and tail.

4

Finally, the spermatids undergo a series of structural changes that transform them into mature **spermatozoa**, or sperm.

Hormonal control and sexual development

Both the testes and the adrenal glands produce male sex hormones, called androgens. These include testosterone, leuteinizing hormone, and follicle-stimulating hormone.

Testes

Adrenal glands

Androgens (male sex hormones)

Testosterone
- Responsible for the development and maintenance of male sex organs and secondary sex characteristics
- Required for spermatogenesis
- Directly affects sexual differentiation in the fetus

LH
- Directly affects secretion of testosterone

FSH
- Directly affects secretion of testosterone

Androgens are responsible for the development of male sex organs and secondary sex characteristics.

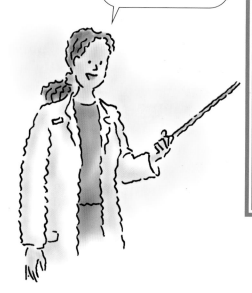

Male secondary sexual characteristics

- Distinct body hair distribution
- Skin changes (such as increased secretion by sweat and sebaceous glands)
- Deepening of the voice
- Increased musculo-skeletal development

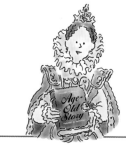

Age-old story

Age-related male reproductive changes

- Decreased testosterone production, which can cause:
  - decreased libido
  - softening and atrophy of the testes
  - reduction in sperm production by 48% to 69% between ages 60 and 80
- Enlargement of the prostate gland
- Diminished prostate secretions
- Decreased volume and viscosity of seminal fluid
- Slower and weaker physiologic reactions during intercourse

Female reproductive system

The female reproductive system consists of external and internal genitalia.

Female external genitalia

The external genitalia, collectively called the *vulva*, consist of the mons pubis, labia majora, labia minora, clitoris, vaginal opening, urethra, and Skene's and Bartholin glands.

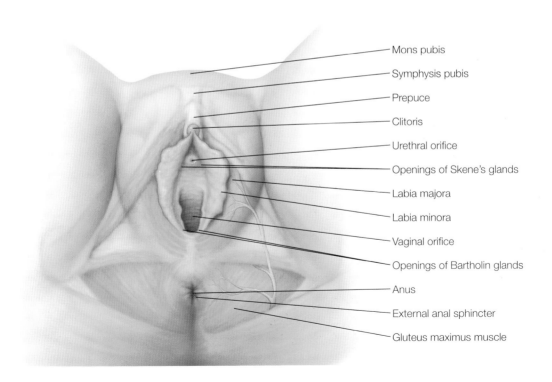

Mons pubis

Symphysis pubis

Prepuce

Clitoris

Urethral orifice

Openings of Skene's glands

Labia majora

Labia minora

Vaginal orifice

Openings of Bartholin glands

Anus

External anal sphincter

Gluteus maximus muscle

Female internal genitalia

The internal genitalia include the vagina, uterus, ovaries, and fallopian tubes.

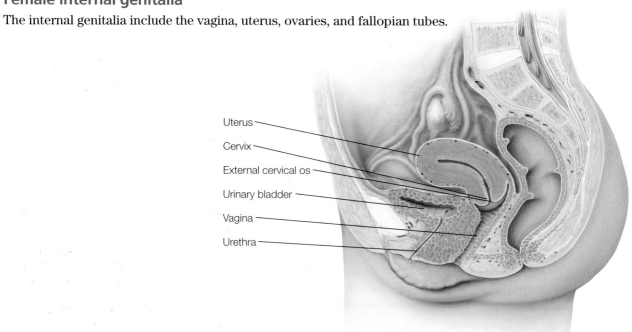

- Uterus
- Cervix
- External cervical os
- Urinary bladder
- Vagina
- Urethra

Ovary, fallopian tube, uterus, and vagina

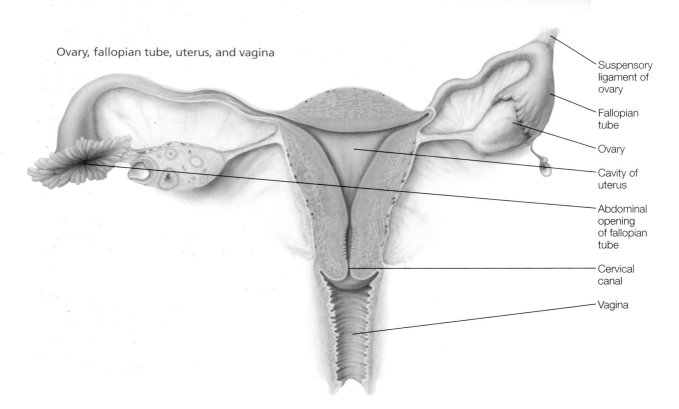

- Suspensory ligament of ovary
- Fallopian tube
- Ovary
- Cavity of uterus
- Abdominal opening of fallopian tube
- Cervical canal
- Vagina

Mammary glands

The mammary glands, located in the breast, are specialized accessory glands that secrete milk.

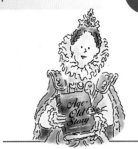

Age-old story

Age-related female reproductive changes

As estrogen levels decrease and menopause approaches, usually at about age 50, changes affect most parts of the female reproductive system.

■ Ovulation stops 1 to 2 years before menopause.

■ Ovaries atrophy and become thicker and smaller.

■ Vulva atrophies, exposing sensitive area around the urethra and vagina to abrasions and irritations.

■ Vagina atrophies and becomes thin and dry, making it susceptible to abrasion. Vaginal pH becomes more alkaline, increasing the risk of vaginal infections.

■ The uterus shrinks until it reaches one-fourth its premenstrual size.

■ The cervix atrophies and no longer produces mucus for lubrication.

■ In the breasts, glandular, supporting, and fatty tissues atrophy. Cooper's ligaments lose their elasticity and breasts become pendulous.

■ Relaxation of the pelvic support commonly occurs, causing pressure and pulling sensations in the area above the inguinal ligaments, lower backaches, and difficulty rising from a sitting position.

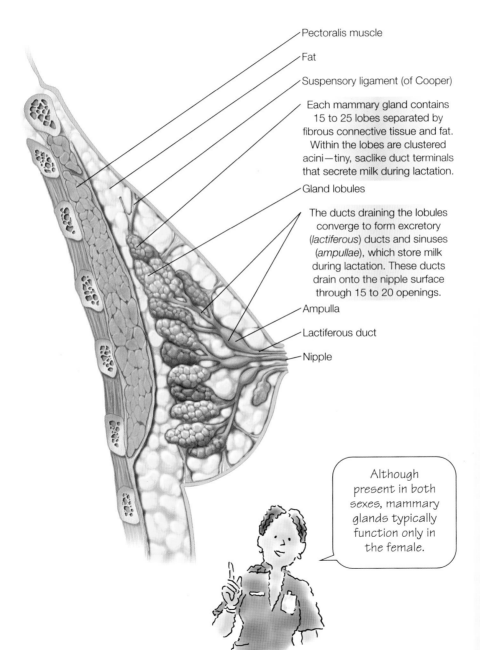

Pectoralis muscle

Fat

Suspensory ligament (of Cooper)

Each mammary gland contains 15 to 25 lobes separated by fibrous connective tissue and fat. Within the lobes are clustered acini—tiny, saclike duct terminals that secrete milk during lactation.

Gland lobules

The ducts draining the lobules converge to form excretory (*lactiferous*) ducts and sinuses (*ampullae*), which store milk during lactation. These ducts drain onto the nipple surface through 15 to 20 openings.

Ampulla

Lactiferous duct

Nipple

Although present in both sexes, mammary glands typically function only in the female.

Hormonal function and the menstrual cycle

When a female reaches the age of menstruation, the hypothalamus, ovaries, and pituitary gland secrete hormones—estrogen, progesterone, FSH, and LH—that affect the buildup and shedding of the endometrium during the menstrual cycle.

During adolescence, the release of hormones causes a rapid increase in physical growth and spurs the development of secondary sex characteristics. This growth spurt begins at approximately age 11 and continues until early adolescence, or about 3 years later.

> The female reproductive cycle is comprised of three different cycles, all working together: ovarian, hormonal, and endometrial.

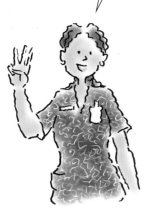

Gonadotropin secretion

Ovarian cycle

- Beginning the first day of the menstrual cycle, low estrogen and progesterone levels stimulate the hypothalamus to secrete gonadotropin-stimulating hormone (Gn-RH).
- In turn, Gn-RH stimulates the anterior pituitary gland to secrete FSH and LH.
- Elevated levels of FSH trigger development of a follicle within the ovary (follicular stage).

- When the follicle matures, a spike in LH level occurs, causing the follicle to rupture and release the ovum, thus initiating ovulation.
- After ovulation (the luteal stage), the collapsed follicle forms the corpus luteum. If fertilization doesn't occur, the corpus luteum degenerates.

Sex hormone cycle

- During the follicular phase of the ovarian cycle, the increasing FSH and LH levels that stimulate follicle growth also stimulate secretion of estrogen.
- Estrogen secretion peaks just before ovulation; this triggers the spike in LH levels, causing ovulation.
- After ovulation, estrogen levels decline rapidly.

- In the luteal phase of the ovarian cycle, the corpus luteum is formed and begins to release progesterone and estrogen.
- As the corpus luteum degenerates, levels of both of these ovarian hormones decline.

Endometrial (menstrual) cycle

- In the first 5 days of the reproductive cycle, the endometrium sheds its functional layer, leaving the deepest layer intact.
- The endometrium begins regenerating its functional layer at about day 6 (the proliferative stage), spurred by rising estrogen levels.

- After ovulation (about day 14), increased progesterone secretion stimulates conversion of the functional layer into a secretory mucosa (secretory stage), which is more receptive to implantation of a fertilized ovum. (The endometrium is most receptive to implantation of a fertilized ovum about 7 days after ovulation.)
- If implantation doesn't occur, the corpus luteum degenerates, progesterone levels drop, and the endometrium again sheds its functional layer (menstruation).

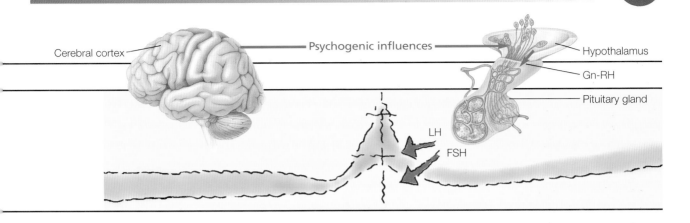

Cerebral cortex — Psychogenic influences — Hypothalamus

Gn-RH

Pituitary gland

LH

FSH

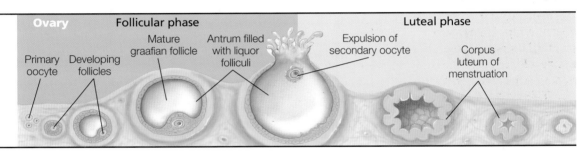

Ovary

Follicular phase

Luteal phase

Mature graafian follicle

Antrum filled with liquor folliculi

Expulsion of secondary oocyte

Corpus luteum of menstruation

Primary oocyte

Developing follicles

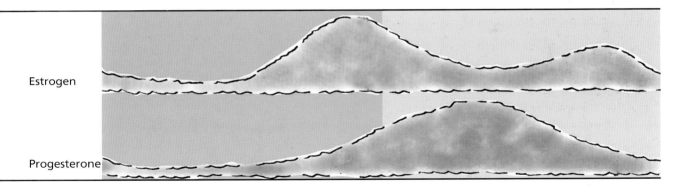

Estrogen

Progesterone

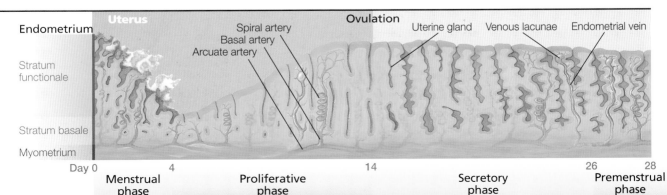

Endometrium

Uterus

Ovulation

Spiral artery

Basal artery

Arcuate artery

Uterine gland

Venous lacunae

Endometrial vein

Stratum functionale

Stratum basale

Myometrium

Day 0   4   14   26   28

Menstrual phase   Proliferative phase   Secretory phase   Premenstrual phase

VISION QUEST

Able to label?

Identify the key structures of the male reproductive system shown in this illustration.

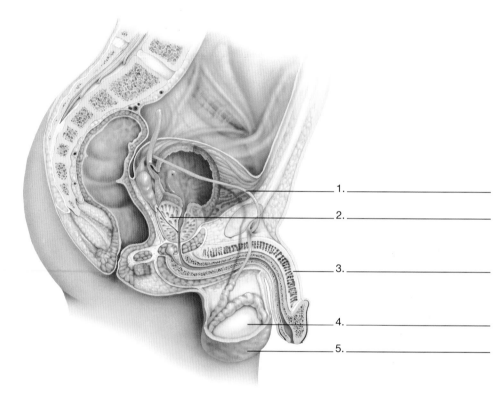

1. _____
2. _____
3. _____
4. _____
5. _____

Rebus riddle

Sound out each group of symbols and letters to reveal information about the male reproductive system.

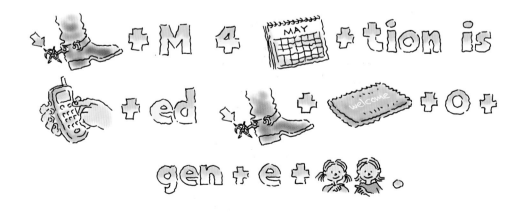

18 Reproduction and lactation

Fertilization 226

Pregnancy 228

Labor and the postpartum period 236

Lactation 241

Vision quest 242

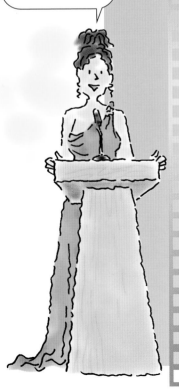

There's no greater production... than the story of reproduction!

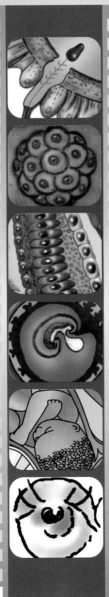

Fertilization

1 The spermatozoon, which has a covering called the *acrosome*, approaches the ovum.

2 The acrosome develops small perforations through which it releases enzymes necessary for the sperm to penetrate the protective layer of the ovum before fertilization.

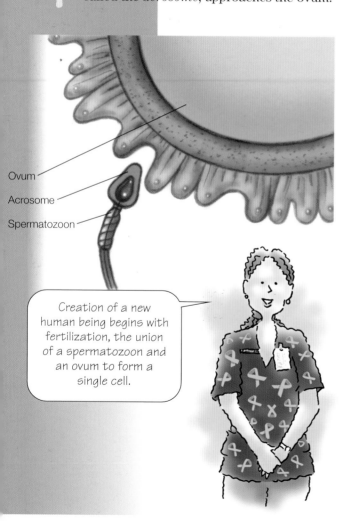

Ovum

Acrosome

Spermatozoon

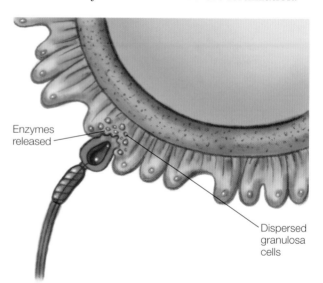

Enzymes released

Dispersed granulosa cells

> Creation of a new human being begins with fertilization, the union of a spermatozoon and an ovum to form a single cell.

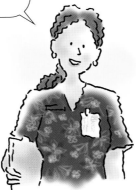

Spermatozoa can survive in the female reproductive tract for up to 4 days.

3 The spermatozoon penetrates the zona pellucida (the ovum's inner membrane). This triggers the ovum's second meiotic division (following meiosis), making the zona pellucida impenetrable to other spermatozoa.

4 The spermatozoon's nucleus is released into the ovum, its tail degenerates, and its head enlarges and fuses with the ovum's nucleus. This fusion provides the fertilized ovum, called a *zygote*, with 46 chromosomes.

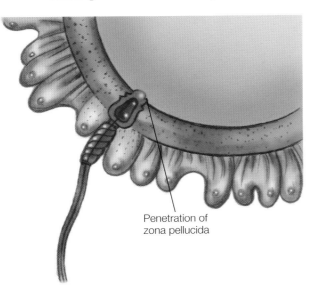

Penetration of zona pellucida

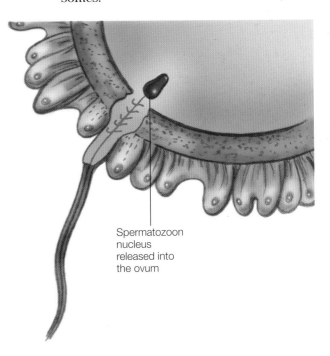

Spermatozoon nucleus released into the ovum

Pregnancy

Pregnancy starts with fertilization and ends with childbirth. During this period (called *gestation*), the zygote divides as it passes through the fallopian tube and attaches to the uterine lining through implantation.

Stages of fetal development

Inside scoop

Pre-embryonic development

Stage	Duration
Pre-embryonic	Fertilization to week 3
Embryonic	Weeks 4 through 7
Fetal	Week 8 through birth

During pregnancy, the fetus undergoes three major stages of development.

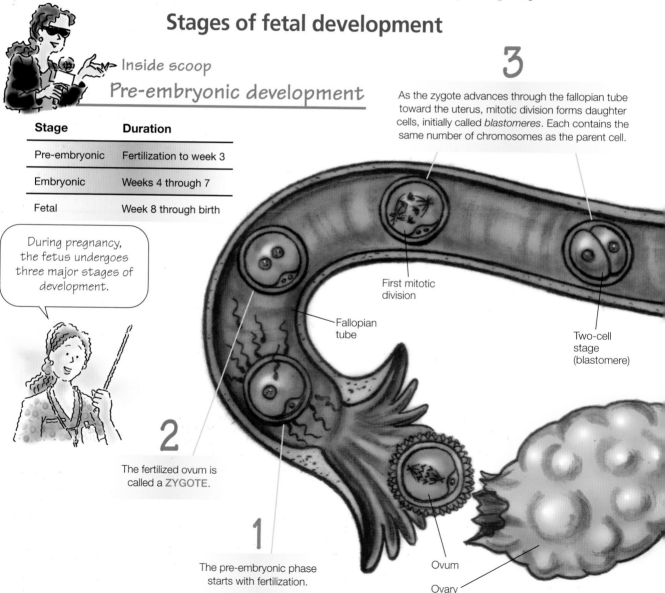

3

As the zygote advances through the fallopian tube toward the uterus, mitotic division forms daughter cells, initially called *blastomeres*. Each contains the same number of chromosomes as the parent cell.

First mitotic division

Fallopian tube

Two-cell stage (blastomere)

2

The fertilized ovum is called a ZYGOTE.

1

The pre-embryonic phase starts with fertilization.

Ovum

Ovary

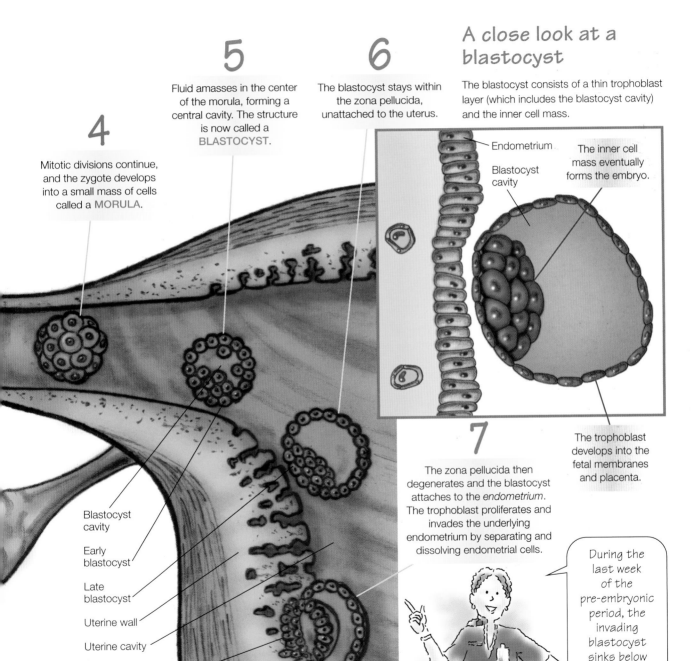

5

Fluid amasses in the center of the morula, forming a central cavity. The structure is now called a BLASTOCYST.

6

The blastocyst stays within the zona pellucida, unattached to the uterus.

A close look at a blastocyst

The blastocyst consists of a thin trophoblast layer (which includes the blastocyst cavity) and the inner cell mass.

4

Mitotic divisions continue, and the zygote develops into a small mass of cells called a MORULA.

Endometrium

Blastocyst cavity

The inner cell mass eventually forms the embryo.

Blastocyst cavity

Early blastocyst

Late blastocyst

Uterine wall

Uterine cavity

Partially implanted blastocyst

7

The zona pellucida then degenerates and the blastocyst attaches to the *endometrium*. The trophoblast proliferates and invades the underlying endometrium by separating and dissolving endometrial cells.

The trophoblast develops into the fetal membranes and placenta.

During the last week of the pre-embryonic period, the invading blastocyst sinks below the surface of the endometrium.

Inside scoop

Embryonic development

During the embryonic period, the developing zygote starts to take on a human shape and is now called an *embryo*. Three germ layers—the *ectoderm*, *mesoderm*, and *endoderm*—eventually form specific tissues and organs in the developing embryo.

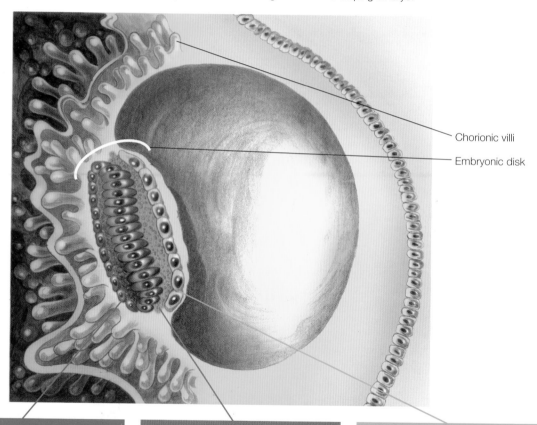

Chorionic villi

Embryonic disk

Ectoderm

The ectoderm, the outermost layer, develops into the:
- epidermis
- nervous system
- pituitary gland
- tooth enamel
- salivary glands
- optic lens.

Mesoderm

The mesoderm, the middle layer, develops into:
- connective and supporting tissue
- the blood and vascular system
- musculature
- teeth (except enamel)
- the mesothelial lining of the pericardial, pleural, and peritoneal cavities
- the kidneys and ureters.

Endoderm

The endoderm, the innermost layer, becomes the epithelial lining of the:
- pharynx and trachea
- auditory canal
- alimentary canal
- liver
- pancreas
- bladder and urethra
- prostate.

Fetal development

Significant growth and development take place within the first 3 months following conception, as the embryo develops into a fetus that nearly resembles a full-term neonate.

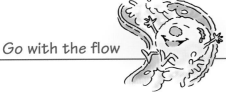

Go with the flow

From embryo to fetus

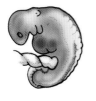

1 month

Month 1

■ The embryo has a definite form.
■ The head, trunk, and tiny buds that will become arms and legs are discernible.
■ The cardiovascular system has begun to function.
■ The umbilical cord is visible.

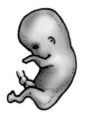

2 months

Month 2

■ The embryo is now called a *fetus*.
■ This month, the fetus grows to 1″ (2.5 cm) in length and weighs 1/30 oz (1 g).
■ The eyes, ears, nose, lips, tongue, and tooth buds form.
■ The arms and legs take shape.
■ The cardiovascular function is complete.
■ At the end of the second month, the fetus resembles a full-term neonate (except for size).

Continued!

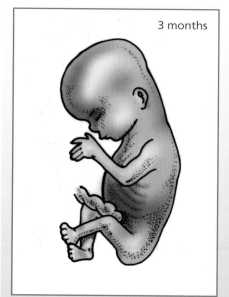

3 months

Month 3

■ This month, the fetus grows to 3″ (7.6 cm) in length and weighs 1 oz (28.3 g).
■ Teeth and bones begin to appear.
■ The kidneys start to function.
■ The fetus opens its mouth to swallow and grasps with its fully developed hands.
■ The sex is distinguishable at the end of the first *trimester* (the 3-month periods into which pregnancy is divided).

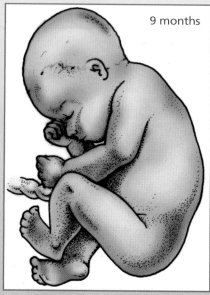

9 months

Months 4 to 9

■ Fetal growth continues as internal and external structures develop at a rapid rate.
■ The fetus stores the fats and minerals it will need to live outside the womb.
■ At birth, the average full-term fetus measures 20″ (51 cm) and weighs 7 to 7½ lb (3.2 to 3.4 kg).

Structural changes in the ovaries and uterus

Specialized tissues support, protect, and nurture the embryo and fetus throughout its development. Among these tissues, the decidua and fetal membranes begin to develop shortly after conception.

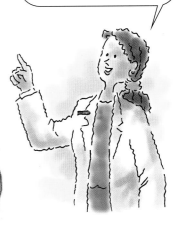

The decidua—which is the endometrial lining during pregnancy—provides a nesting place for the developing ovum.

Approximately 4 weeks

The **decidua basalis** lies beneath the chorionic vesicle.

Chorionic vesicle

Amnion

Yolk sac

The **decidua capsularis** stretches over the vesicle.

The **decidua parietalis** lines the remainder of the endometrial cavity.

Cervix

Vagina

The chorion is a membrane that forms the outer wall of the blastocyst. Vascular projections called *chorionic villi* arise from its periphery.

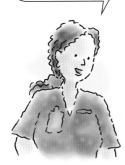

Approximately 16 weeks

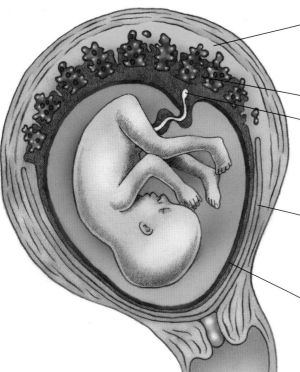

The **chorion frondosum** becomes the rough surface through which the maternal blood flows. Blood begins to flow through this developing network of vessels as soon as the embryo's heart starts to beat.

Decidua basalis

Part of the **yolk sac** is incorporated in the developing embryo, forming the GI tract. Another portion eventually forms oocytes or spermatocytes. During early embryonic development, the yolk sac also forms blood cells. It eventually undergoes atrophy and disintegrates.

The **amniotic sac**, enclosed within the chorion, gradually enlarges and surrounds the embryo. It provides the fetus with a buoyant, temperature-controlled environment. Later, it serves as a fluid wedge that helps open the cervix during birth.

The **chorion laeve** becomes the smooth, inner surface of the placenta.

Placenta

The placenta is flat, pancakelike, and round or oval. The maternal side is lobulated; the fetal side is shiny.

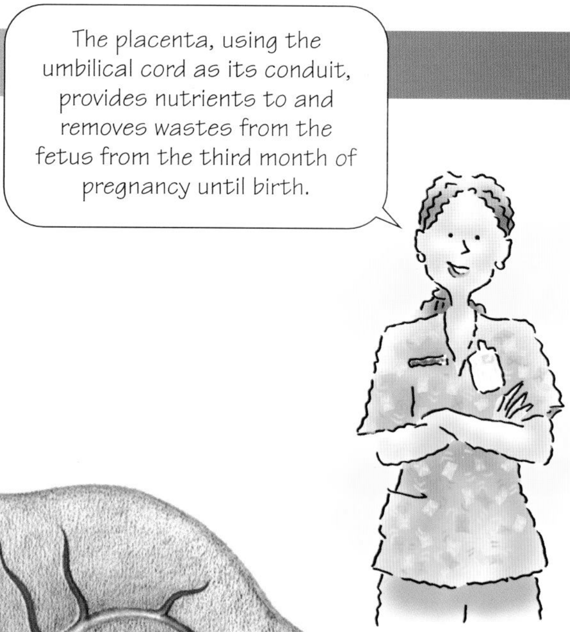

The placenta, using the umbilical cord as its conduit, provides nutrients to and removes wastes from the fetus from the third month of pregnancy until birth.

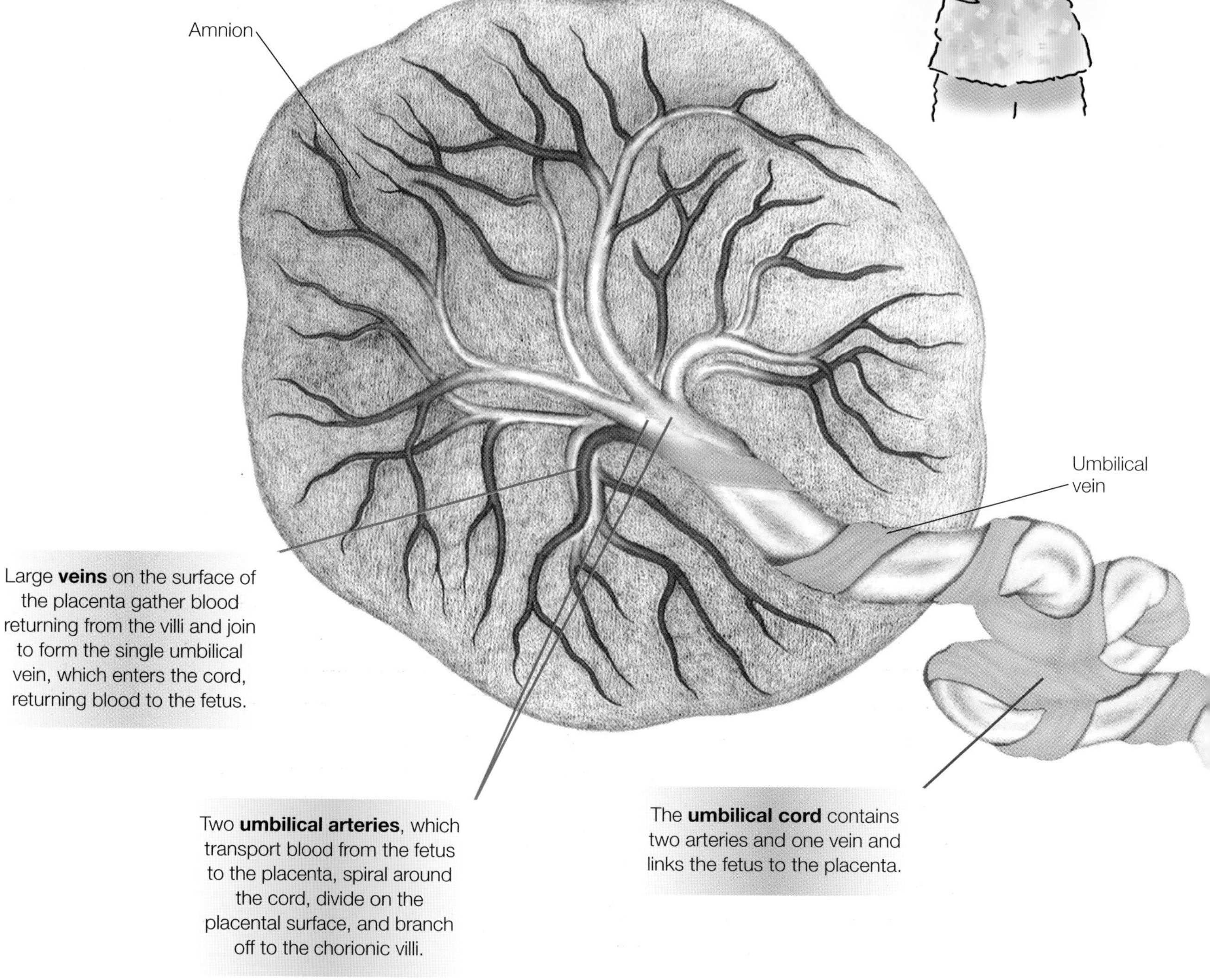

Amnion

Umbilical vein

Large **veins** on the surface of the placenta gather blood returning from the villi and join to form the single umbilical vein, which enters the cord, returning blood to the fetus.

Two **umbilical arteries**, which transport blood from the fetus to the placenta, spiral around the cord, divide on the placental surface, and branch off to the chorionic villi.

The **umbilical cord** contains two arteries and one vein and links the fetus to the placenta.

Types of placental circulation

The placenta contains two highly specialized circulatory systems:

| Uterus | | Placenta | | Fetus |

Uteroplacental circulation

■ This circulatory system carries oxygenated arterial blood from the maternal circulation to the intervillous spaces (large spaces separating chorionic villi in the placenta).
■ Blood leaves the intervillous spaces and flows back into the maternal circulation through veins in the basal part of the placenta near the arteries.

Fetoplacental circulation

■ This system transports oxygen-depleted blood from the fetus to the chorionic villi through the umbilical arteries.
■ It returns oxygenated blood to the fetus through the umbilical vein.

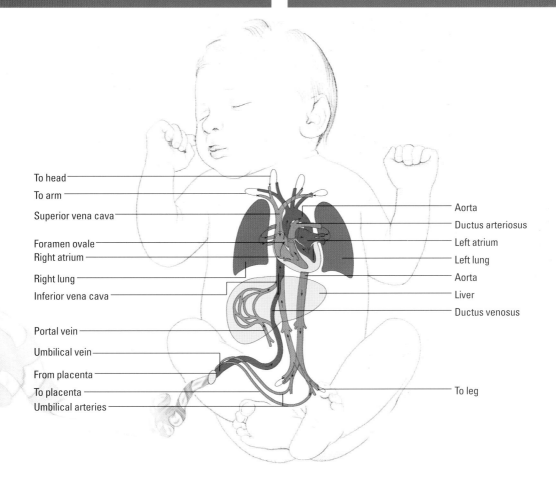

To head
To arm
Superior vena cava
Foramen ovale
Right atrium
Right lung
Inferior vena cava
Portal vein
Umbilical vein
From placenta
To placenta
Umbilical arteries

Aorta
Ductus arteriosus
Left atrium
Left lung
Aorta
Liver
Ductus venosus
To leg

Labor and the postpartum period

Childbirth, or delivery of the fetus, is achieved through labor—the process in which uterine contractions expel the fetus from the uterus. When labor begins, these contractions become strong and regular. Eventually, voluntary bearing-down efforts supplement the contractions, resulting in delivery of the fetus and placenta.

Fetal presentation

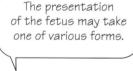

The presentation of the fetus may take one of various forms.

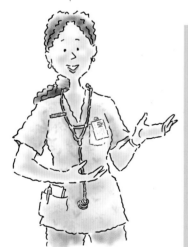

Cephalic

(Head-down presentation)
This position may be classified as:
■ vertex—where the topmost part of the head presents first (shown here)
■ brow or sinciput—where the forward, upper part of the skull presents first
■ face—where the face presents first
■ mentum—where the chin presents first.

Breech

(Head-up presentation)
This position may be classified as:
■ Complete: where the knees and hips are flexed (shown here)
■ Frank: where the hips are flexed and the knees remain straight
■ Footling: where the knees and hips of one or both legs are extended
■ Kneeling: where the knees are flexed and hips extended
■ Incomplete: where one or both hips remain extended and one or both feet or knees lie below the breech

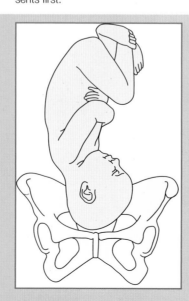

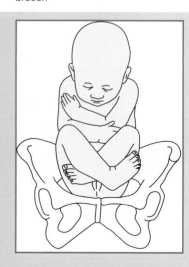

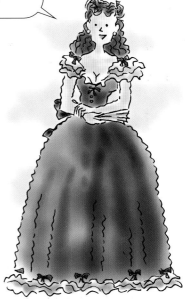

I do declare. It seems that even a fetus understands the importance of making a proper entrance.

Shoulder

(Includes several variations)

■ Because examination can't differentiate among them, all transverse lies are considered shoulder presentations.

Compound

■ Occurs where an extremity prolapses alongside the major presenting part so that two presenting parts appear at the pelvis at the same time.

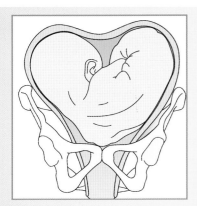

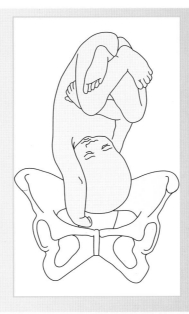

Onset of labor

The onset of labor results from several factors.

■ As the uterus stretches over the course of the pregnancy, nerve impulses stimulate the posterior pituitary lobe to secrete oxytocin (a hormone that stimulates uterine contractions).

■ During pregnancy, the uterus becomes progressively more sensitive to the effects of oxytocin, peaking just before labor onset.

This is it! Stage 1: the onset of true labor.

Stages of labor

The duration of the three stages of labor varies with the size of the uterus, the woman's age, and the number of previous pregnancies.

Stage 1

Hallmark signs of this stage include:

■ cervical *effacement*: the progressive shortening of the vaginal portion of the cervix and the thinning of its walls, and

■ cervical *dilation*: progressive enlargement of the cervical os to allow the fetus to pass from the uterus into the vagina.

The first stage of labor, which lasts until the cervix is completely dilated, is divided into three phases.

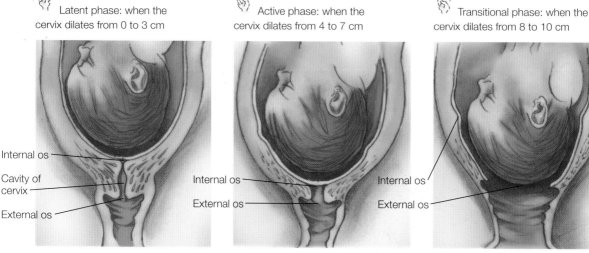

Latent phase: when the cervix dilates from 0 to 3 cm

Active phase: when the cervix dilates from 4 to 7 cm

Transitional phase: when the cervix dilates from 8 to 10 cm

Internal os
Cavity of cervix
External os

Internal os
External os

Internal os
External os

No effacement or dilation

Early effacement and dilation

Complete effacement and dilation

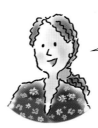

The first stage of labor lasts from 6 to 18 hours in primiparous women and is usually shorter for subsequent births.

Stage 2

The second stage of labor begins with full cervical dilation and ends with delivery of the fetus.

> Short but action packed, the second stage of labor occurs in seven cardinal movements.

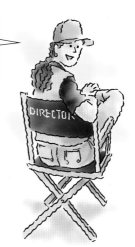

 Engagement, descent, flexion

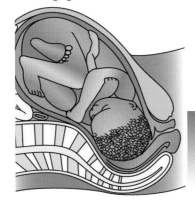

 Internal rotation

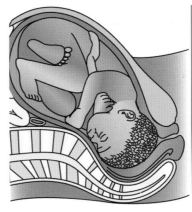

 Extension beginning (rotation complete)

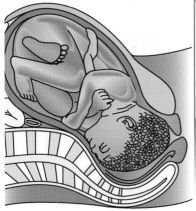

> Continued!

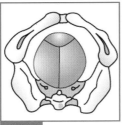

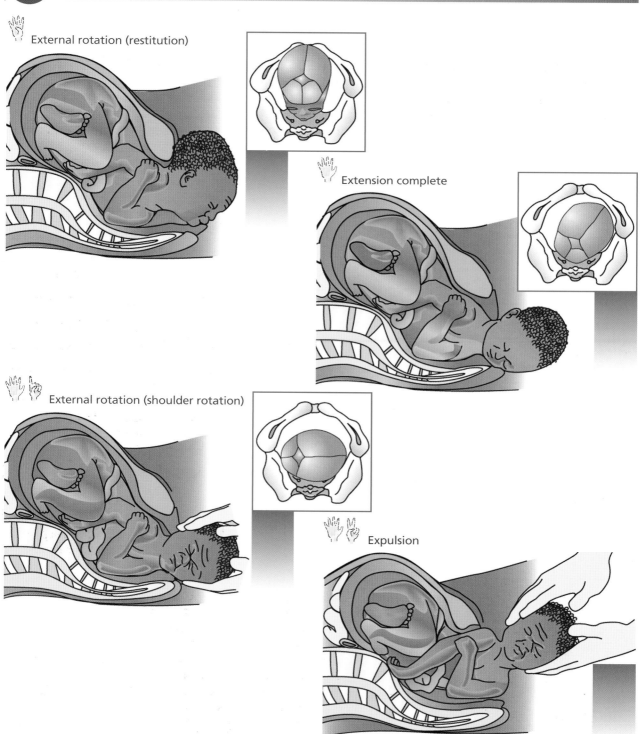

External rotation (restitution)

Extension complete

External rotation (shoulder rotation)

Expulsion

Stage 3

The third stage of labor starts immediately after childbirth and ends with delivery of the placenta.

Postpartum period

After childbirth, the reproductive tract takes about 6 weeks to revert to its former condition in a process called *involution*. The uterus quickly grows smaller, with most of its involution taking place during the first 2 weeks after delivery.

Postpartum vaginal discharge (lochia) persists for several weeks after childbirth.

Lochia rubra

- Consists of a bloody discharge
- Appears 1 to 4 days postpartum

Lochia serosa

- Consists of a pinkish brown, serous discharge
- Occurs from 5 to 7 days postpartum

Lochia alba

- Consists of a grayish white or colorless discharge
- Appears from 1 to 3 weeks postpartum

Uterine involution

After birth, the uterus begins its descent back into the pelvic cavity. It continues to descend about 1 cm per day until it isn't palpable above the symphysis at about 9 weeks after birth.

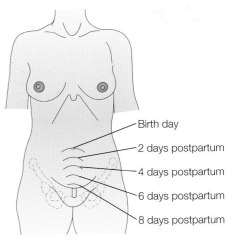

- Birth day
- 2 days postpartum
- 4 days postpartum
- 6 days postpartum
- 8 days postpartum

Lactation

After delivery of the placenta, the body undergoes changes to stimulate the production of milk.

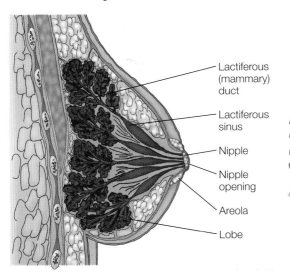

- Lactiferous (mammary) duct
- Lactiferous sinus
- Nipple
- Nipple opening
- Areola
- Lobe

The composition of breast milk changes during the course of a feeding. When a feeding begins, *foremilk* is released. This milk is thin, bluish, and sugary but contains little fat or protein. After the neonate has fed for 10 to 15 minutes, *hindmilk* is formed. This milk is thicker, whiter, and has higher concentrations of fat and protein.

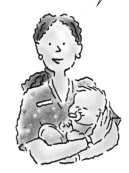

1 First, progesterone and estrogen levels drop, which triggers the production of prolactin.

2 Prolactin stimulates milk production by the acinar cells in the mammary glands.

3 Milk flows from the acinar cells through small tubules to the lactiferous sinuses.

4 When the neonate sucks at the breast, oxytocin is released, causing the nipple to contract and pushing the milk forward through the nipple to the neonate.

VISION QUEST

Show and tell

Using the illustrations here as a guide, describe how fertilization occurs.

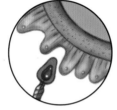 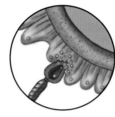 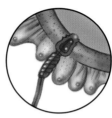 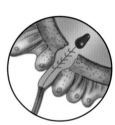

1. _____

2. _____

3. _____

4. _____

_____

_____

_____

_____

_____

_____

Matchmaker

Identify the types of fetal presentation shown here.

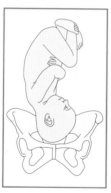 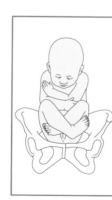 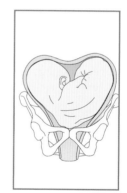 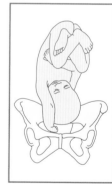

1. _____   2. _____   3. _____   4. _____

A. Breech
B. Shoulder
C. Compound
D. Cephalic

Answers: *Show and tell:* 1. The spermatozoon approaches the ovum. 2. The acrosome develops small perforations through which it releases enzymes necessary for the sperm to penetrate the protective layer of the ovum before fertilization. 3. The spermatozoon penetrates the zona pellucida, triggering the ovum's second meiotic division (following meiosis), making the zona pellucida impenetrable to other spermatozoa. 4. The spermatozoon's nucleus is released into the ovum, its tail degenerates, and its head enlarges and fuses with the ovum's nucleus, producing a zygote. *Able to label?* 1. D, 2. A, 3. B, 4.

Selected references

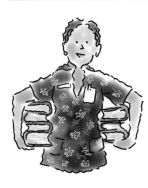

Anatomy & Physiology Made Incredibly Easy, 3rd ed. Philadelphia: Lippincott Williams & Wilkins, 2009.

Assessment Made Incredibly Easy, 4th ed. Philadelphia: Lippincott Williams & Wilkins, 2009.

Bickley, L.S., and Szilagyi, P.G. *Bates' Guide to Physical Examination and History Taking*, 9th ed. Philadelphia: Lippincott Williams & Wilkins, 2006.

Bogart, B.I., and Ort, V. *Elsevier's Integrated Anatomy and Embryology*, St. Louis: W.B. Saunders Co., 2007.

Caughey, A.B., et al. *Blueprints: Clinical Cases in Obstetrics & Gynecology*, 2nd ed. Philadelphia: Lippincott Williams & Wilkins, 2006.

Costanzo, L.S. *BRS Physiology*, 4th ed. New York: Churchill Livingstone, Inc., 2006.

Drake, R., et al. *Gray's Atlas of Anatomy*. St. Louis: W.B. Saunders Co., 2008.

Evans, A.T. *Manual of Obstetrics*, 7th ed. Philadelphia: Lippincott Williams & Wilkins, 2007.

Farquhar, S.L., and Fantasia, L. "Pulmonary Anatomy and Physiology and the Effects of COPD," *Home Healthcare Nurse* 23(3):167-74, March 2005.

Guinan, J.J. "Olivocochlear Efferents: Anatomy, Physiology, Function, and the Measurement of Efferent Effects in Humans," *Ear & Hearing* 27(6):589-607, December 2006.

Hall, J.C. *Sauer's Manual of Skin Diseases*, 9th ed. Philadelphia: Lippincott Williams & Wilkins, 2006.

Jacob, S. *Human Anatomy: A Clinically-Orientated Approach.* New York: Churchill Livingstone, Inc., 2008.

Kasper, D.L., et al., eds. *Harrison's Principles of Internal Medicine*, 16th ed. New York: McGraw-Hill Book Co., 2005.

Monkhouse, W.S. *Master Medicine: Clinical Anatomy*, 2nd ed. New York: Churchill Livingstone, Inc., 2007.

Porth, C.M. *Essentials of Pathophysiology: Concepts of Altered Health States*, 2nd ed. Philadelphia: Lippincott Williams & Wilkins, 2007.

Rubin, E., et al. *Rubin's Pathology: Clinicopathologic Foundations of Medicine*, 4th ed. Philadelphia: Lippincott Williams & Wilkins, 2005.

Seeley, R.R., et al. *Anatomy and Physiology*, 8th ed. New York: McGraw-Hill Book Co., 2007.

Smeltzer, S.C., et al. *Brunner and Suddarth's Textbook of Medical-Surgical Nursing*, 11th ed. Philadelphia: Lippincott Williams & Wilkins, 2006.

Standring, S. *Gray's Anatomy: The Anatomical Basis of Clinical Practice*, 39th ed. New York: Churchill Livingstone, Inc., 2005.

Wahl, I. *Building Anatomy: An Illustrated Guide to How Structures Work.* New York: McGraw-Hill Book Co., 2006.

Credits

Chapter 1

Reference planes, page 3. Willis, M.C. *Medical Terminology: A Programmed Learning Approach to the Language of Health Care*. Baltimore: Lippincott Williams & Wilkins, 2002.

Adipose tissue, page 15, and Types of muscle tissue, page 16. Premkumar, K. *The Massage Connection Anatomy and Physiology*. Baltimore: Lippincott Williams & Wilkins, 2004.

Chapter 7

Taste buds, page 79. Bear, M.F., et al. *Neuroscience: Exploring the Brain*, 2nd ed. Philadelphia: Lippincott Williams & Wilkins, 2001.

Chapter 8

Adrenal glands, page 85. Premkumar, K. *The Massage Connection Anatomy and Physiology*. Baltimore: Lippincott Williams & Wilkins, 2004.

Chapter 11

Inside a lymph node, page 122. Adapted from Eroschenko, V.P. *di Fiore's Atlas of Histology with Functional Correlations*, 9th ed. Baltimore: Lippincott Williams & Wilkins, 2000.

The path of lymph, page 125, illustration 1. Adapted from Cohen, B.J., and Taylor, J. *Memmler's Structure and Function of the Human Body*, 8th ed. Philadelphia: Lippincott Williams & Wilkins, 2005.

Inside the spleen, page 126, illustration 1. Adapted from *Stedman's Medical Dictionary*, 27th ed. Baltimore: Lippincott Williams & Wilkins, 2000.

Chapter 12

Inspiration and expiration, page 144. Weber, J., and Kelley, J. *Health Assessment in Nursing*, 2nd ed. Philadelphia: Lippincott Williams & Wilkins, 2003.

Pulmonary perfusion, pages 146 and 147. Moore, K.L., and Dalley, A.F., II. *Clinical Oriented Anatomy*, 4th ed. Baltimore: Lippincott Williams & Wilkins, 1999.

Chapter 13

Stomach, page 154. Adapted from Cohen, B.J., and Taylor, J. *Memmler's Structure and Function of the Human Body*, 8th ed. Philadelphia: Lippincott Williams & Wilkins, 2005.

Small intestine: How form affects digestion, pages 168 and 169, illustrations 1 and 2. Cohen, B.J., and Taylor, J. *Memmler's Structure and Function of the Human Body*, 8th ed. Philadelphia: Lippincott Williams & Wilkins, 2005.

Small intestine: How form affects digestion, pages 168 and 169, illustration 3. Eroschenko, V.P. *di Fiore's Atlas of Histology with Functional Correlations*, 9th ed. Baltimore: Lippincott Williams & Wilkins, 2000.

Chapter 14

Food group recommendations, page 173. Adapted from U.S. Department of Agriculture, Center for Nutrition Policy and Promotion (2005). MyPyramid Mimi-Poster (Online). Available: *www.mypyramid.gov/downloads/miniposter.pdf*. (2006, September 5).

We also gratefully acknowledge Anatomical Chart Company and LifeART for the use of selected images.

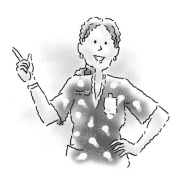

Index

A

Abdominal regions, 5
Accessory lymphoid organs and tissues, 127
Acid-base balance, 211
Acinus, 138
Active transport, 13, 207
Adenoids, 127
Adipose tissue, 15
Adrenal glands, 82, 85
Adrenocorticotropic hormone, 83
Afterload, 101
Agranulocytes, 108, 110, 111
Airflow patterns, 144
Alimentary canal, 152-157, 160-161, 163
    immune function of, 128
    innervation of, 159
    specialized cells in, 155
    structures of wall of, 158
Alleles, 21
Alveolar-capillary membrane, diffusion
        across, 148
Alveolar sacs, 138
Alveoli, 138, 139
Amines, 88
Amino acids, 174, 186, 187
Amniotic sac, 233
Anabolism, 182
Anatomic terms, 2-5
Androgens, 218
Anions, 31, 209
Antibody-mediated immunity, 130
Antidiuretic hormone, 83, 198
Aortic valve, 96, 97
Appendicular skeleton
    bones of, 50, 51
    muscles of, 44, 45
Appendix, 127
Arteries, 102
Arterioles, 102, 146
Arteriovenous circulation, 102-103
Ascending colon, 157
Atom, 27, 28
Atomic structure, 27-30
Atria, 96
Atrioventricular node, 99
Atrioventricular valves, 96, 97
Automaticity, 100
Autonomic nervous system, 69
Autosomal dominant inheritance, 22
Autosomal recessive inheritance, 22
Axial skeleton
    bones of, 50, 51
    muscles of, 44, 45

B

Bartholin glands, 219
Basophils, 108, 110, 111
B-cell formation, 119, 120
Biliary duct system, 161
Bladder, 196
Blastocyst, 229
Blood cells, development of, 108. *See also*
        Red blood cells *and* White blood
        cells.
Blood circulation, 102-103
Blood clotting, 112-114
Blood glucose levels, regulation of,
        184-186
Blood groups, 115
Blood pressure regulation, renin-
        angiotensin-aldosterone
        system and, 199
Blood-typing and crossmatching, 115
Body cavities, 4
Body fluids
    daily gains in, 202
    daily losses in, 202
    forms of, 205
    intake and output of, 208
    movement of, 206-207
    types of, 203
    weight of, 204
Body regions, 5
Bone marrow, 119
Bones, 50-51
    blood supply to, 52
    classification of, 51
    formation of, 53
    functions of, 52
    remodeling of, 53
Bowman's capsule, 195, 197
Brain
    arteries of, 62
    structures of, 60
Breast, 221
Breathing, mechanism of, 144
Bronchi, 137
Bronchioles, 137, 138
Buccal cavity, 153
Bulbourethral glands, 214, 216
Bursae, 55

C

Calcitonin, 84
Capillaries, 102
Carbohydrates, 32, 174
    digestion and absorption of, 179
Cardiac cells, characteristics of, 100
Cardiac conduction, 99-100

Cardiac output, 101
Cardiac sphincter, 154
Cardiovascular system, 94-105
    age-related changes in, 105
    metabolism of, 182-183
Carina, 137
Cartilage, 54
Catabolism, 182
Catecholamines, 85
Cations, 31, 209
Cecum, 156, 157
Cell-mediated immunity, 130
Cells, 6-13
    components of, 6-7
    movement within, 12-13
    protein synthesis and, 8
    reproduction of, 9-11
Central lymphoid organs and tissues,
        119-121
Central nervous system, 60-67
    hormone regulation and, 90
Cerebral lobes, 61
Chemical bonds, 30
Chemical reactions, 29
Chemotaxis, 131
Childbirth, 236
Cholecystokinin, 162
Cholesterol, 175
Chorion, 233
Chorionic villi, 233
Chromosomes, 20
Chyme, 164
Cilia, 135
Clavicle, 143
Clitoris, 219
Coagulation factors, 114
Collecting tubule, 195
Complement system, 131
Compounds, 27
    inorganic, 31
    organic, 32-33
Conchae, 135
Conductivity, 100
Connective tissue, 15
Contractility, 100, 101
Coronary arteries, 104
Coronary veins, 104
Covalent bond, 30
Cowper's glands, 214, 216
Cranial nerves, 68
Crypts of Lieberkühn, 167

D

Dead-space ventilation as cause
        ventilation-perfusion mismatch, 149
Deamination, 187

Decidua, 233
Decomposition, 29
Deep tendon reflexes, eliciting, 66
Defecation, 165
Deoxyribonucleic acid, 8, 9
Depolarization-repolarization cycle, 100
Dermatome, 68
Dermis, 36-37
Descending colon, 157
Diffusion, 12, 148, 206
Digestion, 155, 164-165
   of carbohydrates, 179
   of fats, 181
   of proteins, 180
Digestive enzymes, 86
Dilation, 238
Directional terms, 2
Disaccharides, 174
Distal convoluted tubule, 195
Duodenum, 156, 163

E

Ears, 76-77
   hearing loss and, 76
Effacement, 238
Electrolyte balance, 209-210
   osmotic regulation of sodium and water
      in, 210
Electrolytes as inorganic compounds, 31
Electrons, 28
Electron-transport chain, 182, 183
Elimination, 165
Embryonic development, 230-231
Endocardium, 95
Endocrine system, 82-91
   age-related changes in, 91
Energy, 26
Eosinophils, 108, 110, 111
Epicardium, 95
Epidermis, 36-37
Epididymis, 214, 215
Epithelial cells, types of, in small intestine,
      168, 169
Epithelial tissue, 14-15
Erythrocytes. See Red blood cells.
Esophagus, 153
Estrogen, 88
Ethmoidal sinus, 135
Exchange as chemical reaction, 29
Excitability, 100
Expiration, 144
External respiration, 144-148
Extracellular fluid, 203, 204
   electrolyte composition in, 209
Extrinsic pathway, clotting and, 113

Eyes
   age-related changes in, 74
   extraocular structures of, 72
   intraocular structures of, 73, 74, 75
   muscles of, 72

F

Fallopian tubes, 220
Fats, 15, 175
   digestion and absorption of, 181
Fat-soluble vitamins, 176, 177
Feedback mechanism, hormone regulation
      and, 89
Female reproductive system, 219-223
   age-related changes in, 221
Fertilization, 226-227
Fetal development, stages of, 228-232
Fetal presentation, forms of, 236-237
Fetoplacental circulation, 235
Fight-or-flight response, 69
Filtration, 13
Flatus, 165
Fluid balance, 202-208
   age-related changes in, 204
Follicle-stimulating hormone, 83, 218
Food group recommendations, 173
Frontal sinuses, 135
Fruits, daily recommendations for, 173

G

Gallbladder, 163
Gas exchange, respiration and, 145-148
Gastric inhibitory peptides, 162
Gastric secretion, sites and mechanisms
      of, 167
Gastrin, 155, 162
Gastrointestinal hormones, 162
Gastrointestinal system, 152-169
   age-related changes in, 169
   components of, 152-158, 160-163
   functions of, 164-169
Gastrointestinal tract. See Alimentary
      canal.
G cells, 155
Gene expression, 21
Genes, 21-23
Gestation. See Pregnancy.
Glands, 82-88
Glial cells, 59
Glomerular filtration, 197
Glomerulus, 195, 197
Glucagon, 86
Glucocorticoids, 85
Gluconeogenesis, 184
Glucose catabolism, 182, 183
Glycogen, conversion of glucose to, 184,
      185, 186

Glycogenesis, 184, 186
Glycogenolysis, 184
Glycolysis, 182, 183
Gonads, 88
Grains, daily recommendations for, 173
Granulocytes, 108, 110, 111
Growth hormone, 83

H

Hair, 40
Hearing loss, 76
Heart
   blood flow through, 98
   conduction system of, 99
   location of, 94
   structures of, 95-97
Heart muscle, circulation to, 104
Hematologic system, 108-115
   age-related changes in, 109
Hematopoiesis, 108, 119
Hemostasis, 112-114
Hormones
   classification of, 88. See also specific
      hormone.
   menstrual cycle and, 222-223
   regulation of, 89, 90
   release of, 89, 90
   role of, in blood glucose regulation, 186
   sexual development and, 218
   urinary system and, 198-199
Host defenses, 129
Humoral immunity, 130
Hydrogen bond, 30
Hydrolysis, 179
Hypertonic fluid, 205
Hypothalamic–pituitary–target gland axis,
      hormone release and, 90
Hypothalamus, effect of, on endocrine
      activities, 83
Hypotonic fluid, 205

I

Ileocecal valve, 156
Ileum, 156, 157
Image perception and formation, 75
Immune responses, 130
Immune system, 118-131
   functions of, 128-131
   structures of, 118-127
Inflammatory response, 129
Inorganic compounds, 31
Inspiration, 144
Insulin, 86
   effect of, on blood glucose level, 186
Intake and output of fluid, 208
Integumentary system, 36-41
   age-related changes in, 41

Internal respiration, 144
Interstitial fluid, 203, 204
Intestinal glands, 168, 169
Intracellular fluid, 203, 204
    electrolyte composition in, 209
Intravascular fluid, 203, 204
Intrinsic cascade system, 113
Ionic bond, 30
Isotonic fluid, 205

J

Jejunum, 156, 158
Joints, 54-55

K

Kerckring's folds, 167
Ketone bodies, 188-189
Kidneys, 192-195
    urine formation and, 197
Krebs cycle, 182, 183

L

Labia majora, 219
Labia minora, 219
Labor
    onset of, 238
    stages of, 238-240
Lactation, 241
Lactic acid, blood glucose regulation and,
    185
Laminar airflow, 144
Large intestine, 157
Laryngopharynx, 136
Larynx, 136
Leukocytes. *See* White blood cells.
Ligaments, 49
Limbic system, 61
Lipids, 32, 175
    metabolism of, 188-189
Lipogenesis, 184
Liver, 160
    blood glucose regulation and, 184
    circulation to, 105
Lochia, 241
Loop of Henle, 195
Lower airways, 137-139
Lungs, 140
Luteinizing hormone, 83, 218
Lymph, 123
    path of, 124
Lymphatic vessels, 123-125
Lymph nodes, 122, 125
Lymphocytes, 108, 119

M

Macrophages, phagocytosis and, 131
Male reproductive system, 214-218
    age-related changes in, 218
Male secondary sexual characteristics, 218
Mammary glands, 221
Manubrium, 143
Matter, 26
Maxillary sinus, 135
Meats, daily recommendations for, 173
Mediastinum, 142
Meiosis, 11
Melanocyte-stimulating hormone, 83
Melatonin, 87
Memory cells, 120
Meninges, 67
Menstrual cycle, hormonal function and,
    222-223
Metabolism, 172, 182-189
Milk, daily recommendations for, 173
Mineralocorticoids, 85
Minerals, 176, 178
Mitosis, 10
Mitral valve, 96, 97
Molecule, 27
Monocytes, 108, 110, 111
Monosaccharides, 174
Mons pubis, 219
Motilin, 162
Motor neural pathways, 65
Mouth, 79, 153
Multifactorial inheritance, 22
Muscle fibers, 46
Muscles, 44-45
    age-related changes in, 47
    attachment of, 47
    functions of, 49
    growth of, 47
    movements of, 48
    role of, in blood glucose regulation, 185
    structure of, 46
Muscle tissue, 16
Musculoskeletal system, 44-55
Myocardium, 95

N

Nails, 40
Nasopharynx, 135
Nephron, 194-195
Nerve tissue, 17
Nervous system, 58-69
    age-related changes in, 60
Neural pathways, 65
Neuroglia, 59
Neuron, 17, 58-59
Neurotransmission, 59
Neutrons, 28

Neutrophils, 108, 110, 111
Nose, 78
    immune function of, 128
Nucleic acids, 33
Nutrition
    age-related changes in, 189
    components of, 172-178

O

Olfactory receptors, 78
Opsonization, 131
Oral cavity, structures of, 153
Organic compounds, 32-33
Oropharynx, 136
Osmosis, 12, 207
Ovaries, 88, 220
    structural changes in, during pregnancy,
        233
Oxytocin, 83

PQ

Pancreas, 82, 86, 163
Parasympathetic nervous system, 69
Parasympathetic stimulation of alimentary
    canal, 159
Parathyroid glands, 84
Parathyroid hormone, 84
Parotid gland, 153
Passive transport, 12
Penis, 214
Pericardial fluid, 95
Pericardium, 95
Peripheral lymphoid organs and tissues,
    122-127
Peripheral nerves, 68
Peripheral nervous system, 68-69
Peristalsis, 159, 164
Peyer's patches, 127
pH, 211
Phagocytes, 119
Phagocytosis, 131
Pharynx, 153
Phospholipids, 175
Photosynthesis, 174
Pineal gland, 87
Pinocytosis, 13
Pituitary gland, 82, 83
Pituitary–target gland axis, hormone
    release and, 90
Placenta, 234
    circulatory systems in, 235
Plasma, 109
Plasma cells, 120
Platelets, 112
    development of, 108
Pleura, 141
Pleural cavity, 141

Polypeptides, 88
Polysaccharides, 174
Postpartum period, 241
Pre-embryonic development, 228-229
Pregnancy, 228-235
Preload, 101
Progesterone, 88
Prolactin, 83
Prostate gland, 214, 216
Protective surface phenomena, 128
Proteins, 33, 174
    digestion and absorption of, 180
    metabolism of, 186-187
Protein synthesis, cells and, 8
Protons, 28
Proximal convoluted tubule, 195, 197
Pulmonary arteries, 146-147, 148
Pulmonary function, age-related changes
    in, 142
Pulmonary perfusion, 146-147
Pulmonary veins, 146-147, 148
Pulmonic valve, 96, 97
Purkinje fibers, 99
Pyloric sphincter, 154, 163
Pyruvic acid
    blood glucose regulation and, 185
    lipid metabolism and, 188

R
Receptors, 91
Rectum, 157
Red blood cells, 109
    development of, 108
    life span of, 109
Reference planes, 3
Reflex arc, 63
Reflex responses, 66
Renin-angiotensin-aldosterone system, 199
Respiratory system, 134-149
    age-related changes in, 142
    structures of, 134-143
Respiratory tract, immune function of, 128
Reversible chemical reaction, 29
Rh typing, 115
Ribonucleic acid, 8
Ribs, 143

S
Salivary glands, 153
Saturated fatty acid, 175
Scapula, 143
S cell, 155
Scrotum, 214
Sebaceous glands, 41
Secretin, 155, 162
Semilunar valves, 96, 97
Seminal vesicles, 214, 216

Sensory neural pathways, 65
Sensory system, 72-79
Sexual development, hormonal control
    and, 218
Shunting as cause of ventilation-perfusion
    mismatch, 149
Sigmoid colon, 157
Silent unit as cause of ventilation-
    perfusion mismatch, 149
Sinoatrial node, 99
Sinuses, 135
Skene's glands, 219
Skin
    functions of, 38-39
    layers of, 36-37
Small intestine, 156
    digestion and absorption and, 168
Sodium-potassium pump, 13
Somastatin, 86
Spermatogenesis, 217
Sphenoidal sinus, 135
Spinal cord, 63-64
Spleen, 126-127
Splenic pulp, 126
Stem cells, 119, 121
Sternum, 143
Steroids, 88
Sterols, 175
Stomach, 154
Stroke volume, 101
Subcutaneous tissue, 36
Sublingual gland, 153
Submandibular gland, 153
Suprasternal notch, 143
Surfactant, 139
Swallowing, mechanism of, 166
Sweat glands, 41
Sympathetic nervous system, 69
Sympathetic stimulation of alimentary
    canal, 159
Synthesis, 29

T
Target cells, 91
Taste buds, 79
T-cell formation, 119, 121
T cells, 87
Tendons, 49
Testes, 88, 214, 215
Testosterone, 88, 218
Thermoregulation, skin and, 39
Thoracic cage, 143
Thoracic cavity, 142
Thymus, 87, 119
Thyroid gland, 84
Thyroid-stimulating hormone, 83
Thyroxine, 84

Tissue, 14-17
Tonsils, 127
Trachea, 136, 137
Transamination, 187
Trans fats, 175
Transitional airflow, 144
Transverse colon, 157
Tricuspid valve, 96, 97
Triglycerides, 175
Trigone, 196
Triiodothyronine, 84
Tubular reabsorption, urine formation and,
    197
Tubular secretion, urine formation and,
    197
Turbinates, 135
Turbulent airflow, 144

U
Umbilical cord, 234
Unsaturated fatty acid, 175
Upper airways, 135-136
Ureters, 192, 196
Urethra, 196, 214, 215, 219
Urinary system, 192-199
    age-related changes in, 195
    components of, 192-196
    hormones and, 198-199
Urinary tract, immune function of, 128
Urine formation, 197
Urine output, 197
    antidiuretic hormone and, 198
Uterine involution, 241
Uteroplacental circulation, 235
Uterus, 220
    structural changes in, during pregnancy,
    233-234

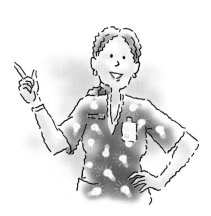

V

Vagina, 220
Vaginal opening, 219
Vas deferens, 214, 215
Vegetables, daily recommendations for, 173
Veins, 102
Ventilation, 144
Ventilation-perfusion mismatch, 148-149
Ventilation-perfusion ratio, 148-149
Ventricles, 96
Venules, 102, 147
Vermiform appendix, 156, 157
Vertebral column, 143
Visceral peritoneum, 158
Vitamins, 176-177
Vulva, 219

W

Water as inorganic compound, 31
Water-soluble vitamins, 176, 177
White blood cells, 110
    classifying, 110-111
    development of, 108

X

Xiphoid process, 143
X-linked dominant inheritance, 23
X-linked recessive inheritance, 23

Y

Yolk sac, 233

Z

Zygote, 227, 228, 230

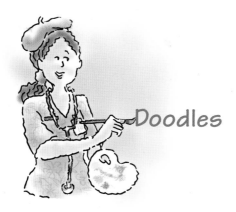

Doodles

Anatomy & Physiology

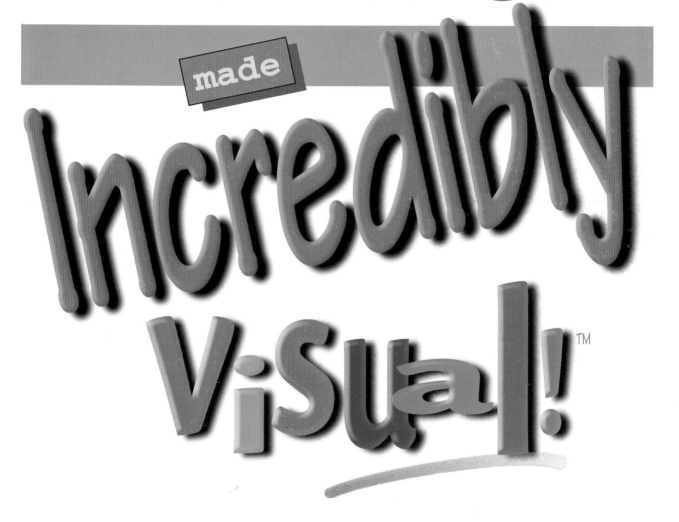

made **Incredibly Visual!**™

 Wolters Kluwer | Lippincott Williams & Wilkins

Health

Philadelphia • Baltimore • New York • London
Buenos Aires • Hong Kong • Sydney • Tokyo

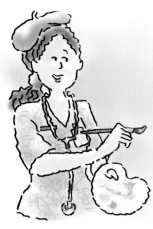

Staff

Executive Publisher
Judith A. Schilling McCann, RN, MSN

Editorial Director
David Moreau

Clinical Director
Joan M. Robinson, RN, MSN

Art Director
Mary Ludwicki

Senior Managing Editor
Jaime Stockslager Buss, MSPH, ELS

Clinical Project Manager
Beverly Ann Tscheschlog, RN, BS

Editor
Gale Thompson, RN, BA

Copy Editors
Kimberly Bilotta (supervisor), Scotti Cohn,
Shana Harrington, Dorothy P. Terry, Pamela
Wingrod

Designer
Lynn Foulk

Illustrator
Bot Roda

Digital Composition Services
Diane Paluba (manager), Joyce Rossi Biletz,
Donna S. Morris

Associate Manufacturing Manager
Beth J. Welsh

Editorial Assistants
Karen J. Kirk, Jeri O'Shea, Linda K. Ruhf

Indexer
Barbara Hodgson

A&PIV010308

Library of Congress Cataloging-in-Publication Data

Anatomy & physiology made incredibly visual.
   p. ; cm. — (Incredibly visual)
   Includes bibliographical references and index.
   1. Human anatomy — Atlases. 2. Human physiology — Atlases. 3. Human anatomy — Handbooks, manuals, etc. 4. Human physiology — Handbooks, manuals, etc. I. Lippincott Williams & Wilkins. II. Title: Anatomy and physiology made incredibly visual. III. Series.
   [DNLM: 1. Anatomy — Atlases. 2. Anatomy — Handbooks. 3. Physiological Processes — Atlases. 4. Physiological Processes — Handbooks. QS 39 A5355 2009]
   QM25.A488 2009
   612.0022'3 — dc22
   ISBN-13: 978-0-7817-8686-7 (alk. paper)
   ISBN-10: 0-7817-8686-X (alk. paper)
                                    2007049049